CANCER
Busters

Paths to
Health
Healing
and
Inner
Peace

Eddie Fitzgerald

D0905990

TWENTY-THIRD PUBLICATIONS
BAYARD 🔵 Mystic, CT 06355

Uncredited quotes and all Scripture translations by the author.

First published (December 1999) by
SDB Media,
St. Teresa's Road,
Dublin 12
Ireland

CancerBusters is an SM of Eddie Fitzgerald and SDB Media.

Twenty-Third Publications/ Bayard
185 Willow Street
P.O. Box 180
Mystic, CT 06355
(860) 536-2611
(800) 321-0411

ISBN:1-58595-093-9
Library of Congress Catalog Card Number: 00-131386
Printed in the U.S.A.

Dedication

For Dr. David Fennelly
and his medical team who are
dedicated professionals and caring people,
for helping to keep me alive
and functional during this time.
Also for all those in the medical profession,
in the hospice movement,
and in the other caring professions
who commit themselves on a daily basis
to those placed in their care.
Without them,
none of us would be as good as we are.
May all of you be blessed with
health, inner peace, and much, much love.

Contents

Cancer Busters

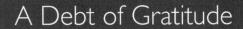

A Debt of Gratitude

No matter how independent we think we are, we don't go through life on our own. Whether we realize it or not, other people play a significant role in our development and growth.

One of the key life strategies in this book is to be willing to ask for help. Many of us are too shy, proud, or even ashamed to do so. When we learn to overcome our fears and ask for help, we may be surprised to find how generous people are with their responses.

All of this is by way of saying that I owe a deep debt of gratitude to many people. Without their professional, technical, and personal support and encouragement, this book might not now be in your hands. If anything in it helps you, touches you deeply, or enables you to get on with your life in a more positive fashion, please remember that the following had a big part to play in it.

For their professional and technical advice, assistance, and practical generosity I am deeply indebted to: Helen Doyle and Gerry Clarke (Impress); Sean O'Boyle (The Columba Press); Bernard Treacy (Dominican Publications); Neil and Pat Kluepfel (Twenty-Third Publications); John Hayes, Gerry Hutchinson, and Basilio Ustarez (Pallas Printing Ltd.); Alex and Aidan Tarbett (Cathedral Books); Maurice Curtis (Veritas); and Sharon Conway (ColourBooks Ltd.).

For their personal support and encouragement I will forever be in the debt of my family and friends: Liam and Anne Fitzgerald, Éilís Bergin, Howard and Mollie Knight, Mick and Ethnea Cummins, Jim and Marjaliisa Betts, Marie Hopkins, Bosco and

John Carroll, Mary and Gerard Cheyrou-Lagreze, Elizabeth
Murphy, Margaret Horgan, Mary Murphy, Kitty and Timmy Ring,
Maureen and Timmy Cronin, Tom and Mairead Murphy, Diana
and Alan Clayton, John Horan, Michael Smyth, Helen Grimes,
Clodagh Putt, Teresa Bradshaw, Anne O'Regan, Marie Campion,
Denis and Carol Bergin, Myles O'Reilly, Betty Foley, Patricia Finn,
Mary and Josephine Sullivan, Theresa and John Hutchinson,
Maureen Bergin, Hannah and Joseph Hutchinson, Teresa
Kennedy, Geraldine and Paddy Armitage, Gloria Taylor, Clarence
Thomson, Dominic McEvoy, Fabio Attard and the S.P.Y.S. team
(Malta), Chris Cullander, Jack Labanauskas and Andrea Isaacs.

I want to acknowledge, too, that we all stand on the shoulders
of giants. I have learned much from the personal contact, teach-
ings, and writings of so many brilliant men and women that it's
not possible to name them all. But I must include the following
who have been crucially significant in my own journey of discov-
ery: Dr. Bernie Siegel, Dr. Howard Benson, Dr. Deepak Chopra,
Dr. Joan Borysenko, Dr. Robert Buckman, Dr. Carl Simonton, Dr.
William Glasser, John Bradshaw, Henri Nouwen, Richard Rohr, M.
Scott Peck, Gerald May, Thich Nhat Hanh, William Johnston,
Robert Wicks, Helen Palmer, Laleh Bakhtiar, Anthony de Mello,
John Shea, Wanda Nash, Richard Carlson, John-Roger and Peter
McWilliams.

In a special way I want to thank my own Salesian Community
in Dublin, who have been so supportive of me during my illness
and the writing of this book: Jim O'Halloran, P.J. Healy, Flor
McCarthy, Pierce Kearns, John Foster, Tom Dunne, Patrick
Brewster, Alan Mowles, and Denis Bowman.

My G.P., Dr. Stephen Ryan, has quite literally saved my life several times with his timely interventions. I owe him a deep debt of
gratitude. I also want to thank John Hyland, Kay Aspil, and our
own loyal staff—Pauline McDonnell, Betty Fogarty, Mary Doyle,

Kay Fogarty, Susan McNally, Phyllis Hoary, Desmond Swinburne, and Oliver Brady.

Special thanks are due to my fellow patients in the hospital who so generously shared their stories and their lives with me, and gave me permission to use them if I thought they would help. Also thanks to all those who have been praying for me since they learned of my condition.

Finally, as in the dedication, I want to thank Dr. David Fennelly and his team and all the medical, nursing, and care staff, especially Dr. Michael O'Leary and nurses Angela Cox and Deirdre McDonnell, for helping to keep me alive and functional during this time, and for their unstinting dedication to all the patients in their care. Indeed, without the commitment and skills of the medical, nursing, and caring professions, and the hospice movement, none of us would be as good as we are. To one and all: health, happiness, and much, much love.

December 1, 1999
Eddie Fitzgerald, SDB
Salesian House, St. Teresa's Rd., Dublin 12

Please Note

This book is meant as a support for people with cancer or other serious illness. It is not intended to be an alternative to proper medical treatment or the recommendations of your doctor and medical team. It is my earnest desire that the material in this book will support their work. If, however, there ever appears to be a conflict between anything in this book and the advice of your doctor, it is vital that you follow your doctor's recommendations. Your doctor knows your individual medical condition and is best *trained* to give you the information you need to deal with it.

IF YOU OR SOMEONE YOU CARE ABOUT HAS BREAST CANCER

You can get help—everything from the latest medical information to emotional support—from the following:

- **National Alliance of Breast Cancer Organizations** at 1-888-806-2226 or *www.nabco.org* on the Web.
- **Susan G. Komen Breast Cancer Foundation** at 1-800-462-9273 or *www.breastcancerinfo.com*.
- **The Y-ME National Breast Cancer Organization** at 1-800-221-2141 or *www.y-me.org* on the Web.

Also, for information on a wide range of breast-cancer concerns—including testing, treating and coping with the disease—call the National Cancer Institute's Cancer Information Service at 1-800-422-6237 or visit *http://www.cancernet.nci.nih.gov/cancer_types/breast_cancer.shtml* or use your :CueCat scanner to swipe the following cue:

C 01 00 00 04 00 09 26

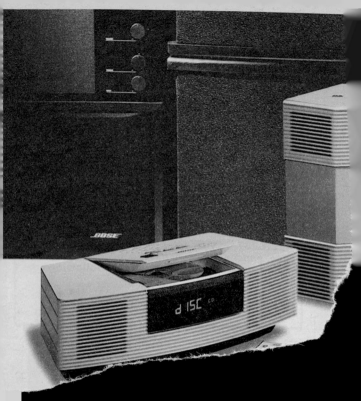

Up Close and Personal

*Life is not a matter
of holding good cards,
it's playing a poor hand well.*
—Robert Louis Stevenson

There's a delightful incident in the life of Mahatma Gandhi which has been very helpful to me. There was a woman who was at her wit's end because of the bad behavior of her young son. The final straw came when he started to smoke before his tenth birthday. In desperation she took him to see Gandhi and said:

"Gandhi ji, I want you to tell my son to stop his bad behavior, be respectful to his mother, and give up smoking."

"Why do you not tell him yourself, daughter?"

"Because he will not listen to me. He respects no one but you. Please, Gandhi ji, help me. Please tell him to stop smoking. If he doesn't, he'll end up just like his father, with lung cancer."

"Come back in two weeks and we'll see," said Gandhi.

"But, Gandhi ji, you could tell him now and we wouldn't have to make the extra journey," replied the woman, the tears rolling down her cheeks.

"I'm sorry," said Gandhi. "There's nothing more I can do today."

The woman and her son left, but two weeks later the two of them returned and stood before the great man. Gandhi put his hand on the boy's head and gently said:

"I want you to stop your bad behavior, to be a good son to your mother and to stop smoking."

"I will, Gandhi ji," replied the boy, his eyes lighting up at being spoken to by his hero.

The woman was delighted and asked the boy to leave while she thanked Gandhi. But when they were alone she couldn't resist the question:

"Surely you could have told him that on our first visit. Why did we have to wait till now?"

"Because, daughter, two weeks ago I myself was a smoker."

The Personal Touch

Nothing is more powerful than personal experience. There are too many people who are over-generous with their advice and suggestions but who themselves do not practice what they preach. To them we rightly say: "Physician, heal thyself."

This book has been written out of lived experience. In my fifty-nine years on this earth I have experienced six different hospitals with everything from broken bones, ulcers, and phlebitis to thrombosis, pulmonary embolism, and now advanced cancer. As my friend Helen put it: "You've been there, done that, and you're wearing the T-shirt!"

There is nothing in this book that I've not tried to practice in my own life. The writing of it has been both therapeutic and humbling, and I share what I have learned with you, hoping you'll find one or two strategies, techniques, or tools that may help you in your own journey through life.

When I was writing it, I was very conscious of all the people who, like me, had been diagnosed with cancer. But I was also thinking of those people who had other serious illnesses, as well as their families, friends, and colleagues. Even nurses, doctors, and consultants may find something in here that might help them in the care of their patients. In other words, the insights outlined in these pages are transferrable to any life, not just to somebody who may or may not have a life-threatening illness.

I've done my best to make it an easy read, something you can pick up at any point, dip into, and come back to later when you have a little more time.

I love stories, and haven't hesitated to tell my favorites. When I worked for a television station I loved being able to share stories with people and left it up to them to discover their own meaning. I firmly believe that only when you discover something for yourself does it become significant in your own life. Remote-control living and hand-me-down platitudes are no substitute for personal enlightenment.

I think we ought to read only the kind of books that wound and stab us. A book must be an axe for the frozen seas within us.
—Franz Kafka

A Learning Experience

"Truth is something you stumble into when you think you're going someplace else." I was reminded of Jerry Garcia's insight when I was told I had advanced colorectal cancer, with metastases on the liver and that its extent was such that it was inoperable. At that moment my whole life was turned upside down.

I had been travelling in one direction and now had to face the prospect of going in another. But in the process I learned more about myself and more about the beauty, dignity, generosity, and goodness of other people than I had in all my years of living before. For that I am grateful to God.

Being Irish, and loving everything to do with words, I want to join in the sentiments and prayer of the old Irish monk who wrote the following at the end of a long hard task:

"My hand is weary from writing; my sharp quill is not steady; as its tender tip spits its dark, blue stream, the words which are formed on the page are jagged and uncertain.

"O Lord, may it be your wisdom, not my folly, which passes through my arm and hand. May your words take shape upon the page. For when I am truly faithful to your dictation, my hand is firm and strong. Let me never write words that are callous or profane. Let your priceless jewels shine upon these pages."

2   Your First Reactions Are Normal

There are no incurable diseases,
only incurable people.
—Dr. Bernie Siegel

When a doctor, surgeon, or oncologist tells you that you have cancer, most people find that it's like a tidal shock-wave hitting them, numbing and stunning them, leaving them initially with almost no feelings at all. The shock to the system is so profound that it frequently leads to disbelief and denial.

There's no need to be surprised at this. It's a perfectly normal defense mechanism. It's one of the ways the mind has of coping with what's happening to the body. It's a way of giving ourselves space in which to take in what is undoubtedly one of the most life-changing events we're ever likely to experience. It's a way of coping with the shock, confusion, fear, anger, and other emotions we naturally experience on being told that we have a very serious and possibly life-threatening illness.

Respect Your First Reactions
This phase will take its own time to play itself out. How long depends very much on the inner and outer resources people have at their disposal. But if we're ever going to start the healing process, it's vital that we are able to get beyond the denial and face the reality of our situation. We're only fooling ourselves if we continue trying to pretend that this is just not happening. More importantly, if we continue to do so, the healing process will nev-

er begin.

Another reaction most people experience is: *Why Me?* This can be a mixture of self-pity and the righteous outrage that seeks to find someone or something to blame.

When I was told I had advanced cancer, I went through all the normal reactions.

Having discovered for myself the lumps on my liver, I tried to face reality and figure out what it might be. My bottom-line was that I might have liver cancer. But I never bargained for the fact that the primary cancer was in my colon.

After all, I'd done all the right things: I didn't smoke, I almost never drank alcohol, I ate plenty of fresh fruit and vegetables, I exercised every day, I confined myself to chicken and fish and avoided coffee and tea. So, what had I done to deserve this? Why me? Well, why not? The truth about cancer is that it is no respecter of persons, even those who do the right things.

Why me? is frequently a subtle form of looking for a scapegoat. We feel the need to identify who or what is to blame and we often begin with ourselves. When we find no real answers there, we may attempt to "shoot the messenger."

I remember being very angry with the surgeon who found the cancer because a year before, with a similar procedure, he had discovered nothing abnormal. It was only when I learned that, in its early stages, cancer is very difficult to detect, that I was able to stop trying to pin the blame on someone else.

Trying to apportion blame is self-defeating. In trying to find someone or something to blame (cigarettes, pesticides, exhaust fumes, radiation, food additives, and genetically modified crops to name but a few) we are effectively giving away our own power. If we are ever going to cope with a serious illness like cancer, we need to retain what power we do have.

Express Your Emotions

Anger is a powerful emotion associated with finding out we have a serious illness. It can be directed against ourselves or others. In my case, it was against others. I was absolutely furious when I learned the full extent of what I had from a piece of paper rather than from another human being.

I've been in the communications business all my adult life and have even lectured on the subject at a university. I know that real communication is not what I say, but what you hear me say. I'm also aware that a diagnosis of cancer is a major shock to the system, and that when we're in shock we can't think straight.

But I told everyone I wanted to know the bottom line. Essentially I'm a practical person. I want to know the whole story; I don't want partial information. Once I know what I'm up against, I can begin to deal with it. However, those who were looking after me thought it best not to give me the bad news all at once, possibly thinking that I couldn't cope with it. It was only the following day, when I read through the text of the clinical trial I had been asked to participate in, that I discovered I had advanced cancer and that its extent was such that it was inoperable.

> *Patience is needed with everyone, but first of all with ourselves.*
> —St. Francis de Sales

When I read that, I hit the roof. I was so angry for the rest of the day that I couldn't rest even with the aid of a sleeping pill.

Eventually, I got up at 4 a.m. and went into the bathroom for a shower.

"Wash all this anger away, Lord," I cried, scrubbing myself with grim determination to get rid of every last vestige of my seething rage, letting the flowing water heal my troubled spirit.

I stayed there for a long time, praying and crying, until my anger began to dissipate and the determination to sort out the situation took over. Having expressed what I felt, I actually felt better. At least now, I told myself, I could get on with my healing. As it happens, the following day I did sort it out with some straight talking with the doctors.

We do ourselves no favors when we try to bottle up our emotions. We need to get them out, to express them in forceful but appropriate ways. Only when we do this will the healing process truly begin.

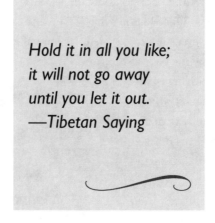

Hold it in all you like;
it will not go away
until you let it out.
—Tibetan Saying

3   It's OK to Feel Afraid

*Bad news goes about in clogs,
good news in stockinged feet.*
—*Welsh Proverb*

Fear is a perfectly normal human emotion. It helps us deal with life in so many ways. It can be positive when it stops us getting too close to the edge of a precipice. But it can also be negative when it prevents us from doing something worthwhile because we're too timid to assert ourselves.

We cannot disrespect our fears. They're real and they're present. They need to be dealt with, but they cannot be downplayed or trivialized. Those who have experienced fear in their lives will know instantly whether people who mouth pious nostrums know what they are talking about or not. It's too easy to say glibly that we should face our dragons and they will then vanish into thin air.

Anyone who has heard the words "I'm sorry to have to tell you, but you've got cancer," will know what fear is. The very word "cancer" still has the power to "frighten us to death" and put us into an emotional tailspin. As Arnold Hutschnecker so forcefully pointed out: "cancer is despair experienced at the cellular level." Media reports on cancer are frequently couched in such negative terms that it's no wonder we have all been conditioned to expect the worst.

It's vital to our healing that we learn how to deal with and calm our fears. As we go through the book I'll present a number

13

of techniques for doing just that. For now it's enough to acknowl-edge that we are afraid, frightened, or even terrified and that that's OK. Indeed, it's to be expected.

There are many reasons why we experience fear. We may be afraid of the prospect of facing a serious operation, of having to deal with chemotherapy or radiotherapy, of watching how all this affects our loved ones, of losing our job through continued ill-health. Most of all, perhaps, we may be afraid of the prospect of dying, sooner rather than later. All of these are legitimate reasons for fear.

Express Fears Openly

It's important that we give ourselves permission to express our fears openly. Studies have shown that there is a definite relation-ship between our ability to express our emotions and the development of cancer. Pretending that every-thing is just fine, when in reality it's not, is a recipe for trouble.

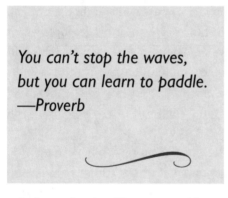

You can't stop the waves, but you can learn to paddle.
—Proverb

We cannot just side-step fear as if it didn't exist. That would be like ignoring the dragon in our living room, in the vain hope that it will go away without seeing us or burning down our house. When we try to hide our fears or hide from them, we are only giving ourselves a temporary respite. Until we begin to accept them and learn to deal with them we won't be able to begin the healing process. Instead, our fears will just reinforce our feelings of helplessness and our inability to cope, and so prevent us from taking the necessary steps to get well.

It's going to be a difficult step to face our fears. And we cannot rush the process. We may even need the help of others to get started. But when we do, we'll find that we may have more power over them than we originally thought possible.

Have no fear for what tomorrow may bring.
The same loving God who cares for you today
will take care of you tomorrow and every day.
God will either shield you from suffering
or give you unfailing strength to bear it.
Be at peace, then, and put aside all
anxious thoughts and imaginations.
—St. Francis de Sales

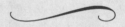

Our Deepest Fear

Our deepest fear is not
that we are inadequate.
Our deepest fear is
that we are powerful beyond measure.
It is our light, not our darkness,
that most frightens us.
We ask ourselves,
"who am I to be brilliant,
gorgeous, talented and fabulous?"

Actually, who are you not to be?
You are a child of God.
Your playing small doesn't serve the world.
There's nothing enlightened about
shrinking so that other people
won't feel insecure around you.

We were born to make manifest
the Glory of God that is within us.
It's not just in some of us;
it's in everyone.
And as we let our own Light shine,
we unconsciously give other people
permission to do the same.
As we are liberated from our own fear
our presence automatically liberates others.
*   —Nelson Mandela*

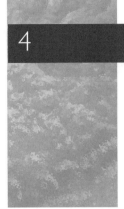

4   Take the First Step

What saves a man is to take a step.
Then another step.
It's always the same step,
but you have to take it.
—Antoine de Saint-Exupéry

A colleague of mine had a catch-phrase that he recommended to anybody who found themselves in a complicated situation that demanded both tact and diplomacy. His advice was: "Whatever you say, say nothing!"

One of the traps we can easily fall into when diagnosed with a serious illness is to temporize. Without realizing it, we can put off taking effective steps towards getting well again. In the initial stages, the shock alone of being hit with the word "cancer" is enough to block any positive move on our part. We can be so stunned by the news that we are unable for the moment to take action. This numbness and inability to act may last a longer or shorter time, depending on our inner resources and how much we're in touch with our true selves.

The Temporizing Trap

It's often when the shock begins to wear off and we're determined to fight, that we're most prone to fall into the temporizing trap. It may be that we're deeply religious. This can lead us to believe that, for some reason, God wants us to have this illness. And there's an element of truth in that. Cancer can be one of the most powerful wake-up calls anybody ever gets. It can put us in touch with what is deepest and most authentic in our lives. It can remind us that we are finite and that our lives are not totally in our own hands.

But we can also adopt a skewed approach to religion. It's one thing to put our trust in God, but divine providence is no excuse for our inaction. After all, "God helps those who help themselves." Five centuries before Christ, the Greek physician Hippocrates put it well when he said: "Prayer is certainly good, but, as people call on the gods, they should themselves lend a hand."

Procrastination Blocks Healing

Another, even more common, way of putting off our healing is through information overload. Knowing more about an illness is a positive thing and will help us deal with it with greater effectiveness. But knowledge on its own will do nothing for us. If we are not careful, we can easily postpone taking any concrete steps to getting better until we have assured ourselves that we have assembled all the information we can about the disease.

It took me nearly five months to realize that this was precisely what I was doing myself. I bought and borrowed every good book I could find on cancer. I read and studied every one of them, making copious notes. I researched the subject in libraries and on the Internet. I investigated conventional medical treatments and complementary remedies. I wanted to inform myself about all the possibilities before I took any determined action.

Meanwhile I was only making half-hearted attempts to bring about my own healing. Since I didn't want to make a mistake, I preferred to do nothing until I was sure of the right way to go. In reality I had adapted my colleague's phrase to my own circumstances: "Whatever you do, do nothing!"

At that point, exercising caution was my motto. This, to me, was the safer and more sensible option. But in effect it was nothing more than a rationalization, a way of avoiding reality. We are easily seduced by illusions when reality is difficult to bear.

Postponing the healing process, for whatever reason, is both short-sighted and ill-advised. What is needed is a multi-track approach.

Trust in the providence of God is a powerful source of healing energy. Finding out more about our disease is extremely helpful in developing healing strategies. But it is vital that we begin right away to take the first steps in implementing some of the practical approaches developed in this book.

When Neil Armstrong first set his size eleven boots on the moon in 1969, he captured the significance of the moment in a memorable phrase: "That's one small step for man; one giant leap for mankind."

What we do right away in our determination to get better may only be a small step, but that in itself can be a giant leap forward in our healing process. Forget my diplomatic colleague and take as your motto: "Whatever you do, do something!" And do it now.

> *There are two mistakes one can make along the road to truth; not going all the way, and not starting.*
> —*Buddha*

God Will Provide!

One winter the rainfall was so heavy that it completely submerged a small town. The local priest was young and healthy and made every effort to help those who were in difficulties. He waded waist-deep in the water, helping out wherever he could. Some aid workers came to his assistance in a little boat but he insisted on carrying on, saying: "God will provide!"

Later, as the water level rose to his chest, another boat came along and he helped get an elderly woman on board, but refused to go himself since, as he intoned with great trust: "God will provide!" Shortly afterwards the water was up to his neck and he had difficulty keeping afloat. This time an air-rescue crew came by in a helicopter and winched two people to safety from a rooftop. When they tried to get hold of the priest he insisted they help somebody else since, as he shouted, "God will provide!"

When they left, the priest eventually got into difficulty and drowned. St. Peter met him at the gates of heaven and showed him in to see God. The priest complained bitterly that he'd done everything he could to help others and yet he himself hadn't been saved. "I put my trust in you, God," he said. "Why didn't you do anything?"

"What do you mean do nothing?" replied God. "Didn't I just send you two boats and a helicopter!"

5   Name It, Claim It, Tame It

The beginning of wisdom is to call things by their right names.
—*Chinese Proverb*

In our stress management workshops through the years, one of the strategies people have found most helpful is: Name It, Claim It, Tame It.

Putting a name on what the problem is or what is causing us concern is vital if we're ever going to come to grips with it. Unfortunately, many people avoid doing so.

> **He:** "I was sorry to hear about John. What did he
>   die of?"
> **She:** "The big 'C'."
> **He:** "I didn't realize he'd drowned."
> **She:** "No, not drowned....you know what I mean—
>   C-A-N-C-E-R."
> **He:** "Oh. Why didn't you say so?"

This exchange, which actually happened, would have been funny had it not been so tragic. The use of the word "cancer" seems to strike such feelings of helplessness, fear, and even terror into people, that they try to find euphemisms for it. They may actually spell the word out—as if they didn't want to be overheard saying it.

We've already noted how our fears paralyze us. This is another example. Most people think so negatively about the prospects of

21

surviving cancer that their terror is projected onto the word itself. But it's important to understand that "cancer" is a word, not a sentence. It's the generic name for a serious illness which may or may not be life-threatening. When we avoid using the word we are effectively reinforcing its negative connotations and making our healing and recovery that much more difficult.

Claim It

The second requirement is to accept it as our own. It's in me, not out there. Acceptance is affirmative and assertive, not compliant and yielding or an act of submission. It's an acknowledgment of reality. Once we accept reality our healing begins. Without such acceptance there can be no healing. All we are likely to experience is worry, anger, depression—in a word, dis-ease.

> *One does not become empowered by imagining figures of light, but by making the darkness conscious.*
> *—Carl Jung*

This was the point which St. Irenaeus was making when he said: "What has not been accepted cannot be redeemed." He was speaking in a religious context, but the principle holds true in all areas of life. It's a central element in the best of modern psychology as well as in religious belief and spirituality. If I do not "own" the condition, I cannot hope to deal with it effectively.

However, claiming something is not the same as identifying with it. The great danger with saying: "I'm a cancer patient. I'm a cancer survivor," is that we invest our identity in our illness. It's vital to remember that our real self is separate from what we're enduring. A more appropriate claim might be: "I'm a person who happens to have cancer. I've also had measles. I'm not my illness. I am much, much more."

When we limit our self-definition to our medical condition, we merely reinforce a negative self-image and this does nothing to help our prospects for recovery.

Tame It

When we learn to give our illness its proper name and accept it as our own, we immediately gain a certain amount of control over it. This is the start we need on the road to healing and inner peace.

In his delightful fable, *The Little Prince*, Antoine de Saint-Exupéry has an insightful passage about the nature of taming. The fox asks the little prince to tame him. When he replies that he doesn't know what "taming" means, the fox points out that it means to establish ties, to take the time to get to know who or what it is you wish to tame.

> *Be willing to have it so; acceptance of what has happened is the first step to overcoming the consequences of any misfortune.*
> —William James

Taming our illness will undoubtedly involve time, effort, and sacrifice. It will also involve a variety of different strategies and resources. But at least we'll be moving in the right direction. Attempting to deny the truth of our situation is only going to delay the process of healing.

A Healthy Self-Image

The Hollywood screen idol, Victor Mature, was as famous for his beefcake physique and impassive expression as for his roles as the biblical hero in *Samson and Delilah,* as one of the leading characters in *The Robe,* and as the gambler in *My Darling Clementine.* He died of cancer aged eighty-six.

Rarely did he seem to do much more than go through the motions on the screen. "There's a lot to be said for loafing, if you do it gracefully," he said.

Those who knew him appreciated his delightfully self-deprecating and laid-back approach to life. He charmed people by not taking himself too seriously. "I have two looks," he would tell his directors. "Do you want Number One or Number Two?"

On one famous occasion, when a pompous secretary of a country club turned him down for membership on the grounds that they didn't accept actors, he famously retorted: "Hell, I'm no actor, and I've got twenty-eight pictures and a scrapbook of reviews to prove it!"

His attitude to life was such that he was in no danger of over-identifying with either his roles or his cancer. He seemed to know intuitively that we are always more than who we say we are, and that labels, compulsions, or diseases can never define our unquenchable spirit.

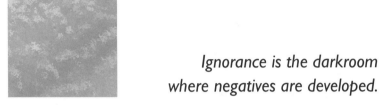

6   Understand What's Happening

Ignorance is the darkroom
where negatives are developed.

Did you know that there are over 200 different cancers and that most of them are eminently treatable? When I was first diagnosed I certainly didn't. It was only when I took the time and trouble to find out more about what I was facing, that I began to see how complex a condition it really is. This, in turn, has helped me deal with it in a realistically positive way. It has given me more possibilities to exercise some control over it and to break its stranglehold on me.

We live in an information age, where those who have access to the knowledge have a definite edge on their competitors. "Knowledge is Power" is their motto.

Some Facts About Cancer
There is a great deal of truth in that, but knowledge is not the be-all and end-all. It's important to realize that knowledge is not understanding—the capacity to perceive the meaning and significance of things. Still less is it wisdom—the capacity to make use of one's experience, knowledge, and understanding in a mature, judicious, and enlightened way. However, it is an essential first step and a great help in dealing with all kinds of issues.

When you've been diagnosed as having cancer, it doesn't necessarily follow that your life is in immediate danger or that there is a medical emergency. A very large number of cancer patients are now being made well again by an ever-expanding variety of modern medical interventions. Numbing and shocking as it is to be diagnosed with cancer, there is still hope for us all. It is true that not everyone will be cured, but it is a fact that everyone can be healed—a distinction well worth keeping in mind.

Cancer is what happens to our body when some of our cells start to replicate uncontrollably. If we only knew what triggers this process and what could shut it down, we'd be in a much better position both to prevent it happening and to treat it when it does.

Risk Factors

Some of the commonest risk factors associated with cancer are smoking, excessive exposure to the sun, a high-fat and low-fiber diet, and a history of the disease in one's immediate family. But why the process starts in the first place is still not fully understood, though researchers are discovering more about it every year. In time this may lead to the vital breakthrough that will allow the medical profession to treat even more cancers successfully.

> *Never mistake knowledge for wisdom. One helps you make a living; the other helps you make a life.*
> —*Sandra Casey*

When you think of the incredible complexity of the human body it's actually little wonder that sometimes things do go wrong. It's estimated that there are about fifty trillion cells in our bodies. Think about it. Not millions, not billions—trillions. The number is simply mind-boggling. Yet when you add to that the fact that each and every one of these cells has a complete set of some three billion genetic bits, you'll quickly appreciate the odds against everything going right all the time. You could say that given the cellular complexity of the human body it's inevitable that mistakes and aberrations will take place.

Whether we are aware of it or not, the cells in our bodies are growing or dying all the time. Every time we visit the hairdresser we acknowledge that fact. Every time we cut our nails or have a manicure, it's because our cells are actively reproducing. In these instances the rate of reproduction is predictable and controlled. When we cut ourselves, our cells respond by accelerating their growth in order to repair any damage caused. Once they have done their job they get a signal to slow down and everything is back to normal again.

The problem with cancer is that some cells are out of control. For whatever reason, when these rogue cells are triggered, they go haywire and keep on multiplying until a primary tumor or lump is formed. Not content with this, they also have the ability to invade surrounding normal tissues, and, by getting into the bloodstream, lymph nodes, and other channels, even to spread to distant parts of the body, creating secondary tumors (metastases).

Different Cancers
This process of uncontrolled growth and invasion is common to over 200 different cancers. But particular cancers behave in different ways. No two are precisely the same. That's why they need different approaches and treatments. Moreover, some cancers are almost never life-threatening, others are potentially lethal, and most of them are somewhere in the middle of the scale.

Many cancers are curable today. There are basically three main forms of treatment: surgery, radiation therapy, and chemotherapy. However, it's worth noting that the medical profession speaks of a "cure" only when there is no evidence of the presence of cancerous cells and when there is no chance of the cancer recurring. Depending on the type of cancer, this may take up to five years to determine, or it may even extend to twenty years or more.

In addition, many cancer patients experience "remission," which is not the same as a cure. Remission can be either partial or complete, depending on whether the tumor has become smaller or whether it is completely undetectable. Some of those who have been successfully treated, or who are in remission due to other interventions, may never experience a recurrence of their cancer. Unfortunately, others may not be so risk-free.

The reality is that, even with cancer, we can still get on with our lives. It's my earnest desire that some of the tools, techniques, and strategies in this book will assist you in doing just that.

> *Still round the corner there may wait*
> *A new road, or a secret gate.*
> —*Alvin Toffler*

7   Remember You're Different

Don't follow the path.
Go where there is no path
and begin the trail.
—Ruby Bridges

Modern science and technology show how different we all are. DNA fingerprinting and retinal scanning are only two examples of how our difference helps to distinguish our uniqueness.

Not only that, but quantum physicists now suggest that our bodies are not as substantial as we once thought. The atoms and molecules that go to make it up are in continuous motion, so much so that scientists speak of it as process rather than a fixed mass of matter. We're different all right. Indeed, each one of us is unique.

All this has important implications for those of us who have serious illness.

Life in a Dressing Gown

My friend Éilís has worked with me for over ten years now, giving workshops and seminars to business, educational, religious, and other professional groups. One of the stories she tells about herself always gets a laugh of recognition.

She was visiting a friend for the weekend and they'd planned to go shopping together. Being a morning person, Éilís was up bright and early. In fact, she was ready to go when the lady and her daughter eventually appeared in their nightgowns and slippers. It took them ages to get themselves sorted out for breakfast and, when they'd finished, they opened a board game and started to play.

Éilís had been waiting patiently all this time, but the board game was the final straw. She decided enough was enough, so she got the keys of the car and said: "I'm off to the shops now. By the time I get back you'll probably have your act together."

To which her friend gently replied: "We have our act together. It's just a different act!"

You Can't Compare Illnesses
Often when we're ill we begin to compare ourselves with others who have a similar illness. If they've got breast or lung cancer we tend to look for the similarities and forget how different we all are.

But it's important to remember that we've all got our own song to sing in life. We've a uniqueness and an individuality which cannot be replicated. Consequently, we respond to illness and treatment in very different ways.

Two people getting the same chemotherapy treatment can have totally different reactions. One may experience a raft of side-effects, while the other sails through it without a bother. Patients who have similar operations recuperate at different rates.

As the old monks used to say: "When you were born, God broke the mold." There will never be another quite like you.

Nowadays most doctors are clued into this and, while they explain to their patients some of the more common side-effects of treatment, they do not go through the whole list in case it becomes a self-fulfilling prophecy.

Apple computers came up with an interesting advertising line some time ago: *Think Different*. Whatever about the grammar, this isn't a bad slogan to have when you're afraid you'll experience the same symptoms or conditions as the next patient. You are the one with the illness, and you'll respond in your own special way. This knowledge can be an integral part of your healing and inner peace.

A Meditation on Being Special

God has created me to do him
some definite service;
He has committed some work to me
which he has not committed to another.
I have my mission;
I never may know it in this life,
but I shall be told it in the next.

I am a link in a chain,
a bond of connection between persons.
He has not created me for naught.
I shall do good, I shall do His work;
I shall be an angel of peace,
a preacher of truth in my own place,
while not intending it,
if I do but keep His Commandments.

Therefore I will trust Him.
Whatever, wherever I am,
I can never be thrown away.

If I am in sickness,
my sickness may serve Him;
in perplexity,
my perplexity may serve Him;
if I am in sorrow,
my sorrow may serve Him,
He does nothing in vain.
He knows what He is about.
He may take away my friends,
He may throw me among strangers,
He may make me feel desolate,
make my spirits sink,
hide my future from me—
still He knows what He is about.
—Cardinal Newman

8   Ask For and Accept Help

When love is involved
no one is a burden.
—Dr. Bernie Siegel

Many people are fiercely independent. No matter how ill they are, they insist on doing things themselves: "It's OK. I can manage," they say. As long as they have a breath of energy, they're determined to use it. I know all about this, because it's my natural style of acting too.

What this effectively amounts to is a form of control—an attempt to remain in charge of our lives, to determine what happens to us. It also gives us permission to forget the fact that our independence is just as problematic as our dependence. Worse still, it means we have never really accepted our interdependence.

Turning the Mattress

I still remember the first time I had to ask someone to help me make my bed.

I was five months into my weekly chemotherapy schedule. Ever since the age of ten, when I got my own room at home, I had been making my bed daily, dutifully turning the mattress once a week, and generally keeping the room tidy. By the time I got to boarding school in my early teens it was second nature to me. Yet here I was, some forty years later, having to ask somebody to help me make my bed because I was no longer able to turn the mattress. I was both ashamed and embarrassed that a piece of bedding could so easily take away my sense of independence. But eventually I asked, and I got immediate help.

When we're ill we have to learn to be humble enough to accept our limitations and ask for help when we need it. The lovely thing is that people are delighted to be asked, and are only too willing to oblige. In fact, it makes them feel good. There is nothing better to boost a person's self-image than the feeling that they are able to give something to another without recompense.

Just think of the number of times in the past when you yourself were able to help out. Not only did it make you feel good about yourself, but somehow it also energized you. The reality is that when we ask others for help, we're providing them with an opportunity to be givers rather than takers, to share rather than hoard, to serve rather than be waited upon. We are offering them a gift which most of them are only too ready to accept.

Learning the Hard Way

About six weeks later I was congratulating myself on having learned the lesson of the bed the hard way. By this time I was able to ask for assistance in turning the mattress and even making the bed without too much embarrassment. However, one morning, when I needed to do some personal shopping, I thought I could kill two birds with one stone. I decided to fulfill two large book orders for city-center bookstores and deliver them in myself.

When I had finished boxing the books, a friend happened to notice that I was a bit out of breath. Immediately, without my prompting him, he said he was going into the city in the afternoon and would be happy to deliver the boxes for me. I thanked him right away, but said that I would probably be all right delivering them myself. As soon as I'd said it, I knew I'd just rejected an act of kindness, but he accepted my short-sighted need for independence gracefully.

It took me a full half-hour to realize that I still hadn't learned the lesson of the bed. Asking for help is only one part of the equation. The other is accepting it when it's offered—even when you didn't ask for it in the first place!

So I went to my friend and said I had been foolish in not accepting his offer. He made it easy for me and took charge of the boxes. Later that morning I was glad he had, because, if I'd attempted to do the deliveries myself, I wouldn't have had the energy to finish my own shopping.

When we learn to ask for help whenever we need it, and accept it whenever it's offered, we'll have gone a long way towards preserving what little energy we have, and giving ourselves a real chance of getting well.

It is one of the beautiful compensations of this life that no one can sincerely try to help another without helping himself.
—Charles Dudley Warner

9   Watch Your Language!

When old words die out on the tongue, new melodies spring forth from the heart.
—*Rabindranath Tagore*

You don't have to be crazy or gaga to talk to yourself. The reality is that we talk to ourselves all the time. In fact, we're so used to doing it that we don't even realize it's happening.

Socrates once said that "the unexamined life is not worth living." Our self-talk is one way of examining our life on a moment-to-moment basis. But what's missing in this exercise is the broader picture.

It has been estimated that some eighty per cent of our self-talk is negative in content. If you pay attention to what you're saying to yourself in any one day you'll find that this is probably about right. We all have a tendency to concentrate on what's going wrong, not on what's going right. We tend to think in terms of problems, mistakes, difficulties, frustrations, and the endless list of negatives that are in everybody's physical, mental, emotional, and spiritual kit bag.

The Power of Words
It's vital for our personal growth and development that we are familiar with the following basic truth: the words we use shape and form our experience.

Words are creative. "In the beginning was the Word" (John 1:1). Words are powerful. If you say: I can't, you're right—you can't. If, instead, you say: I can, you're also right—you can.

36

Words can also reveal attitudes and subvert beliefs. That's why in today's world there is so much emphasis on using inclusive language—words that are non-gender specific and that do not bolster up the dominant position or ideology of one group over another.

When we're seriously ill, the words we use are crucially important. If I had my way I would ban the use of the word "terminal" in connection with cancer. It leads to such negative expectations that it's very likely to become a self-fulfilling prophecy if we don't cancel it out and look at our illness in a different way.

The Double-Cancel Technique

What I call the Double-Cancel Technique is particularly useful when you find yourself thinking or saying something negative. All you have to do is to pull yourself up short with the two simple words Cancel/Cancel. The first cancel is to change the underlying counterproductive thoughts and replace them with more empowering ones; the second is a reminder to wipe out the words you've just used and re-phrase them constructively.

In effect what you're doing is deciding to change your mental tape and put your self-talk into more productive language. This means that from being self-defeating and even destructive, your self-talk can now be beneficial and support you in your healing.

For example, you may find yourself saying (aloud or in your head): "I can't eat salt anymore; the doctor says it's bad for my blood-pressure." As soon as you realize what you've just said, stop yourself immediately by repeating Cancel/Cancel. Then proceed to re-think the thought and re-phrase the words.

The truth of the matter is that you can eat salt, any time you want to. It's just that now you are making a positive choice not to do so based on professional advice and scientific research. So, your re-phrasing might go something like this: "I'm choosing not to take salt right now because my doctor has convinced me that this will help lower my blood-pressure. Having good health is far better than having salted potatoes!"

Her are a few more examples of the technique in practice in the context of being hospitalized or of having a serious illness like cancer.

The Double-Cancel Technique

Negative: I hate being in the hospital.
Positive: I'm glad I'm in a place where they can look after me professionally.

Negative: There's a terrible draught from that window.
Positive: It's good to get some fresh air for a change.

Negative: I'm dying for a bar of chocolate; I need the boost.
Positive: I'm glad I can eat fruit; it's so healthy and gives me the long-term energy I require.

Negative: It took ages for the chemo to arrive this morning!
Positive: Thank God they're taking such care to make sure I get the right dose.

Negative: I hate the sight of those needles and the very thought of them being stuck into me.
Positive: I find that when I take a deep breath and don't look at the needle, I can scarcely feel it going in.

Negative: The pain in my shoulder is a nuisance.
Positive: My body is telling me something with this pain in my shoulder. I'll check it out when the doctor comes.

Negative: I only wish I could do more.
Positive: Small victories are still victories; I'm glad I'm coping as well as I am.

Negative: This whole thing is getting too much for me.
Positive: When the going gets tough, the tough get going!

Negative: Why do I have to face so many problems in my life?
Positive: A challenge like this helps bring out the best in me and will leave me stronger for next time.

Negative: This obstacle seems utterly insurmountable.
Positive: When I can't climb over an obstacle I can generally find a way around it. It may take longer, but I'll still end up on the other side.

10   Conserve Your Energy

*Any fool can be fussy and rid himself
of energy all over the place, but a man
has to have something in him before
he can settle down to doing nothing.*
—J. B. Priestley

My friend Maurice was a great soccer fan. Every year he had a regular ritual. He would travel up to Dublin for the final in September and take in a show the night before. He'd always have somebody to go to the show with, so I was never asked. One year, though, as everybody else was busy, Maurice asked me to take him to see a variety show in the Olympia Theatre. I'd provide the transport, he'd provide the tickets. A more than fair arrangement.

Off we went and thoroughly enjoyed the show. But when we came outside to the car park and I tried to start the car I found that the battery was totally dead. Not a glug, not a splutter. The only explanation I could come up with was that I'd left the lights on when I parked. This simple oversight had drained the battery and left us stranded.

Fortunately, we were able to hail a passing taxi. The driver took out a pair of jumper cables and proceeded to link his battery with ours. Within five minutes of this jump-start we had enough energy stored to get us going, and I gave thanks to God for all Good Samaritans, especially those carrying jumper cables!

Our Energy Tank

The incident with Maurice happened many years ago, but it still reminds me to keep my batteries charged. I'm not talking here

40

about laptops, phones, calculators, and other gadgets. Where the lesson is really important is in making sure that our energy levels are always full, that there is a reserve tank we can access at all times.

When you've got cancer, or indeed any other serious illness, it's vitally important to conserve as much of your energy as possible. If we let our energy supply drain away, or, worse still, actually give it away, we won't be able to access our inner or outer resources, or even be able to muster the motivation to get better.

We've all got a storage tank of energy. Different cultures call it different things. When I did some work in China just over a year ago, I learned a lot about this energy system which courses through our bodies as a life-force. They call it *chi*. It matters little what you call it. The fact is that we all have it.

However, the size of our energy tank varies from person to person. Some seem to have more, some less. But one thing we all share is that our supply of energy is limited. If we fritter it away we become more vulnerable to our illness and its side-effects, and substantially diminish our chances of healing and recovery.

Not that we have to adopt a Fort Knox-type attitude and protect this treasure with armed guards around the clock. If we are ever going to enjoy life, we have to expend our energy. What we're talking about here is not the legitimate use of what's in our storage tank, but the needless loss of a precious and limited resource.

Whenever we find our energy levels running low it's important to do two things:

First of all we need to identify the source of the leakage and plug it. It's vital to know where we expend our energy and why. Without this knowledge we'll never know whether we're going to be in energy credit or debit at the end of the day.

Many things can cause us to lose energy: emotions like anger, frustration, fear, and anxiety are major culprits. So too are relationships, work, and the daily variety of obligations and commitments we are involved in. Whatever is draining our energy must be avoided.

Secondly, we need to get into the habit of plugging into an energy main, a supply source that will continue to top off our daily ration of vitality. This can range all the way from physical exercise and cat naps to visualization and meditation.

Whatever gives us our juice is an important contributor to our well-being and health.

Hold on to Hope

Hope is the thing with feathers
That perches in the soul,
And sings the tune without the words,
And never stops at all.
—Emily Dickinson

When the film *Life is Beautiful* first came out, there was some considerable controversy about the way in which the father tried to protect his son from the horrors of the concentration camp by pretending they were actually playing a game. But what he was doing in reality was striving to hold on to hope, despite the appalling circumstances in which he found himself. He hoped against hope, convinced that even a make-believe hope is better than no hope at all.

Hope is a very real source of energy and a powerful healing force in life. Dr. Bernie Siegel, in his wonderful book *Love, Medicine and Miracles,* makes the point in typically down-to-earth language:

"Let's say I recommended eating three peanut butter sandwiches a day to cure cancer. Some people would get well and claim it was the peanut butter that did it. Then even more people would have hope, eat peanut butter, and get well, too.

"But we know it's not the peanut butter. It's their hope and the changes they produce in their lives while they're on the new therapy."

The Story of the Fork

Hope is a sign of a healthy spirituality, and helps us through even our darkest moments. Fr. Thomas J. McSweeney, the Director of the Christophers, once shared a story that illustrates this beautifully.

Jenny Flanagan was diagnosed with cancer and given three months to live. She decided to put her affairs in order and spoke with her pastor about the details of her funeral service, telling him what Scripture readings and hymns she wanted.

She also told him what she wanted to wear in her coffin. "And this is very important," she added. "I want to be laid out with a fork in my right hand."

The priest didn't know what to say in response, but Jenny explained the situation. "My favorite part of attending church functions and socials over the years was that, when we had a meal and had finished the main course, someone would gently remind me: 'you can hold on to your fork.' I loved that, because I knew something better was coming. I knew then that the dessert was going to be something substantial, and not a watery concoction.

> *God is our refuge and strength: always present to help in times of trouble.*
> —Psalm 46:1

"That's why I want people to see me there in the casket and say: 'What's with the fork?' When they ask you that, you can tell them that I knew that, after the main course, there was always something better to come!"

The lesson of the fork is one of hope and trust. Hope is a virtue that demands effort on our part. It's not something passive, like wishing something would happen but doing nothing about making it happen. It's vibrant and active and demands that we play our part. As the proverb has it: "Trust in God, but row for the shore."

When we truly believe in God's benevolent providence and infinite love, that belief will enable us to hold on to hope and know in our hearts that there's something better still to come. Not even death can quench that kind of hope.

In the face of uncertainty there is nothing wrong with hope.
—Dr. Carl Simonton

12 Deepen Your Spirituality

To live in faith is to see things
always against an infinite horizon.
—Ronald Rolheiser

Many self-help books talk about spirituality as if we all knew what we were talking about. And in a sense we do. But it's worthwhile specifying what we mean before talking about going deeper.

There's a difference between religion and spirituality. One way of looking at it is that religion is for those who want to avoid hell, while spirituality is for those who have been there! Cancer patients, and those who have other serious illnesses, certainly appreciate what this means.

You can, therefore, have a spirituality without belonging to a particular religion. In effect, my spirituality is the daily living out of the beliefs, values, and priorities that I profess to be important in my life. It's the way I live out my life so that my actions match my thoughts and words. It's something that affects every area of my life. It's a style of living, a way of seeing reality whole and of responding to it in love. It expresses itself in every decision I make, and involves both the sacred and the secular dimensions of my life.

Christian spirituality, on the other hand, is the way in which we live out our lives in the here and now in response to the message of Christ and the blessing of the Spirit. It's not confined to prayers and good deeds, but penetrates and animates our every thought, word, and action.

46

Our spirituality is the way we live from our "center," the very core of our being. Many people are content to live on the surface all their lives. They do not go deeper. Indeed, one of the greatest temptations of modern living is precisely that of superficiality— the way in which our culture inclines us towards trivial and distracted living. Spirituality is a way of getting in touch with our center and discovering that God is already present there.

One day during the writing of this book, I lost my spiritual center completely. It happened because of a series of minor catastrophes. One was the complete collapse of my computer monitor and the other was the fact that I had developed phlebitis in both my legs and the pain was excruciating. Anyway, I lost sight of my spiritual center that day.

The following morning, as I was praying just before rising, I was given what I now call "a wisdom gift." It came to me that maybe all the hassle and discouragement I was experiencing might hold a message for me. Maybe it was

Spirituality is how we embody our spirit, incarnate our beliefs, and make real what we profess to hold dear.

God's way of reminding me that I was still trying to do it all myself, that I needed to let others play their part in the production of this book. And, most of all, that it was God's project and not mine. So I prayed for the gift of inner peace, which in my case meant doing my share of the work and then leaving the worry of getting it out on time to God. If God wanted this book published, then let God sort it out! For the rest of that day the burden on my shoulders was much lighter, and I experienced a tranquillity and calm that surprised me.

The burden of cancer can be considerably lightened if we begin to live from our center. In deepening our spirituality, we considerably enhance our ability to deal with our illness and have access to a powerful source of inner healing.

*Spirituality is the way in which we make soul-values present in our world.
It is soul manifesting itself in street clothes.*

The Cancerbuster's Creed

I believe that cancer is a word, not a sentence. Even though it may eventually be the cause of my death, I can live with it successfully and deal effectively with the problems it inevitably brings.

I believe that cancer can be a blessing in disguise—a threshold moment, a wake-up call to put first things first and get my priorities right.

I believe that cancer helps focus my attention on the beauty, wonder, and sheer abundance of creation; that it gives me back the inquiring spirit of childhood when everything was new, everything was fresh, and everything was experienced with surprise and joy.

I believe that cancer helps me appreciate the enduring value of friendship, the comfort of knowing that there are people around who are prepared simply to be present, without the need for any other agenda.

I believe that cancer is an opportunity for family, friends, and colleagues to rally around and offer help in what to them may be down-to-earth and quite mundane ways, but which to me have taken on a significance out of all proportion to their ordinariness.

I believe that cancer helps me discover my spirit, opens me up to the infinite, and puts me in touch with the depths of my soul.

I believe that cancer is a challenge for me to grow up spiritually, and to put into practice the values and beliefs to which I once paid little more than lip service.

I believe that cancer connects me with God, who is present within me, and that this breakthrough moment will forever affect the rest of my life.

I believe that cancer teaches me to be grateful for life, to respect its presence in all its forms, to live each moment as if it were my last, and experience the present to the full.

I believe that cancer gives me the freedom to be who I really am, to say—out of love—what needs to be said, to listen with understanding to another's pain, and to face reality now rather than later.

For the blessing of these beliefs, I daily give thanks to my God.

13   Access Your Inner Resources

*What you bring away
from your illness
depends very much
on what you bring to it.*

Dolly Parton is a true life-force. With her bubbly personality and musical talent, once seen she's never forgotten. Ever since I first saw her I've warmed to her. Her good humor is infectious, her melodies memorable, and her philosophy of life positive.

What makes her so unforgettable, I believe, is her love of life, her total unpretentiousness. Her parents were tough, no-nonsense country folk, trying to bring up their family in the midst of surrounding poverty. She suffered physical abuse and humiliation. Yet she came through it all with her essential spirit intact. She made the best of the cards she had been dealt and went on to fame and fortune through hard work and an unshakable sense of her own value.

Dolly's Patchwork Coat
When her mother gave Dolly a patchwork coat because she was too poor to buy her daughter a new one, Dolly couldn't wait to get to school to show it off. Her mother had reminded her about the Bible story of Joseph and his multi-colored coat, which made his brothers even more envious of him than they already were. But when she got to school, the children made fun of her instead of delighting in her new coat. She was devastated at the time, but later used the experience to write the song *Coat of Many Colors*.

51

When her marriage broke down, Dolly proceeded to pick herself up and get on with life. This time she wrote the stunning *I Will Always Love You*, which became the theme tune of the film *The Bodyguard*. No matter what happens in her life, Dolly seems to have the inner resources to be able to deal with it. She knows how to access these resources so that they become her allies in coping with the "slings and arrows of outrageous fortune" that Shakespeare talks about. As she put it herself: "I took a sad hard time and turned it into a beautiful song."

Optimists and Pessimists

Dolly is a born optimist. She looks on the bright side of life, emphasizes the positive, minimizes the negative, and with determination looks for the silver lining, no matter what kind of cloud attempts to darken her sky.

Two men looked out through prison bars;
One saw mud, and the other saw stars.

Pessimists and optimists are poles apart. Pessimists blame themselves for the difficulties in which they find themselves. Optimists always look for an alternative explanation—their healthy self-image allows them to acknowledge responsibility while refusing to accept that they are wholly to blame.

Pessimists are forever in meltdown mode, locked into thinking of their troubles as being interminable. Optimists keep in mind the dictums that what goes up must come down and this, too, shall pass.

Pessimists are so trapped in negative thinking that they are convinced one mistake leads inevitably to another and that their current difficulties are actually setting them up for future failures. Optimists look at the future as a whole new ball game, where previous performance does not necessarily determine the outcome. Being pessimistic in our approach prevents us from accessing our inner resources. We need to take the optimistic view, and like Dolly Parton, make the most of what we've got and get on with the business of living.

> *The first sign of maturity
> is the discovery
> that the volume knob
> also turns to the left.*
> —*"Smile" Zingers*

14   Avoid Toxic People

*An optimist may see a light where
there is none, but why must the
pessimist always run to blow it out?*
—*Michel De Saint-Pierre*

One of the most common ways of losing energy is to keep company with negative or toxic people.

These come in all shapes and sizes but they have one thing in common. They drain energy from people. They're like vampires who suck the life-force out of us and then move on to their next unfortunate victim.

Life is too short to accept anything but the best. A friend of mine, Michael, suggested how I might express it in more graphic terms. So, I now say: "The sign of a healthy personality is the capacity not to accept Charlie, Roger, Alpha, Piper from anybody!"

The following are just a few of these toxic types. The list is not exhaustive; you'll know many others from your own experience. What matters is that when you come across any of them, you give them a wide berth. Particularly when we are ill we should strive to surround ourselves with positive people and avoid those who steal our energy through their negativity.

Whiners are people who are always moaning about something, who think the world owes them a living and who feel justified in sitting back and complaining about how things are not working out for them.

Manipulators are people who use their native guile to twist us round their little finger and get what they want in the most subtle and covert ways imaginable.

Controllers are people who use their power for their own ends and who force others to do their bidding, employing a variety of techniques from guilt to helpfulness to get what they really want themselves.

Parasites are people who batten on to others, cling to them, profess their neediness and pretend to be helpless so that people will feel sorry for them and give them some of their own energy.

Narcissists are people who are so vain and egotistical that they have fallen in love with their own reflection. They need you to give them an endless supply of praise and admiration to compensate for their hidden feelings of inadequacy.

Pessimists are people who continually see the bottle as half empty and who insist that their negative view of people, situations, and events is just being "realistic."

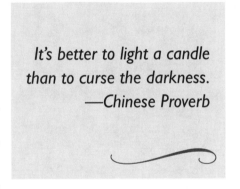

It's better to light a candle than to curse the darkness.
—Chinese Proverb

When you feel your energy draining away, check to see how it's being lost. If it is because you are paying too much attention to toxic people, make the decision now not to invest your limited resources in such a negative venture.

Surround Yourself With Positive People
The natural corollary to all of this is to surround yourself with positive people.

Positive people are those who give you energy, who affirm your efforts, who encourage you to keep going, who praise your small victories, who listen to your tales of woe, who empathize with your pain, and who comfort you when you feel very much alone.

With such people in your life, you can cope better with any setbacks that may arise and enhance your prospects of getting well.

A friend is someone who comes in when the whole world goes out.
—Anonymous

Release Your Creativity

*Creativity cures
the chaos in the heart.*
—Tibetan Proverb

Cancer and other serious illnesses are wake-up calls that cannot be ignored. But there is an aspect of this waking up which is sometimes forgotten. This is a pity, because it can in fact help us in our recovery or, when recovery is not possible, in our spiritual healing and inner peace.

One of the things that happens when we're faced with serious life issues is that, for the rest of our time on earth, we want to live life to the full. That implies getting out of our routines, avoiding the ruts, and beginning to plow new furrows whenever possible. Tilling new soil in our lives becomes a desirable goal.

Creativity on Steroids

When I was first put on steroids to counteract the dreadful exhaustion that the chemotherapy was causing, I was so peppy that every part of my body felt alive and tingling. I slept very little, had enormous energy, and ate like a horse. I regained all the weight I'd lost, and then some! The nausea ceased and I felt absolutely wonderful, on a permanent "high." I understood then why athletes may be tempted to enhance their talents with the aid of drugs.

One day, while I was on a break in London, I took the train to Leicester to visit some friends of mine, Howard and Mollie, who have a farm in the country. During the journey a single line kept flashing through my head: "The man with the wooden leg." My father, long since dead, had only one leg. Ironically, he was the town shoemaker. And I thought, there's something important here that I must do—but what?

That night, comfortable in bed, but unable to sleep, I watched some British Broadcasting Company educational programs for an hour or so, and then the dam burst. I took up pen and paper and wrote a poem in praise of my father—something I wouldn't have dreamt of doing before my illness. I include it in the following pages, not as a sample of good poetry, but as an indicator of what's possible when you let loose your creative juices and sing a new song.

Hidden Potential

I believe there's a divine energy field all around us, enveloping the earth and the entire universe. Nothing exists without it. As a Christian I believe that we are held in the palm of God's hand. But you don't have to believe in God to accept quantum physics. This speaks of an energy field that everything taps into.

Deepak Chopra makes this point beautifully in *Unconditional Life*. He takes the example of a rose. Both the leaf and the thorn are nourished by the same sunlight. Photosynthesis is basically the same in each, and their DNA is identical.

"The difference between a leaf and thorn is a matter of selection," he writes. "The thorn takes sunlight and turns it into something hard, sharp, and pointed. The leaf takes sunlight and turns it into something soft, rounded, and translucent. By itself, sunlight has none of these qualities."

It's an essential part of our ability to create that we can activate our potential by selecting or choosing to do one thing rather than another. Things we once took for granted may now take on a new meaning. Activities we wouldn't have considered in other circumstances now become attractive.

In practice, releasing our creativity can range all the way from writing poetry, learning a foreign language, or enrolling in a painting class, to discovering the pleasures of gardening, cooking, or playing a musical instrument. Whatever floats your boat, do it! Release your hidden potential. It will make you feel vibrant and alive again, and support you when you most need it.

The Man With the Wooden Leg

I remember the man with the wooden leg
as if it were yesterday,
though it is now nearly fifty years ago.

Not that he wore it all that often.
It wasn't supple enough for everyday fare.
He trotted it out on Sundays
concealed in his best suit.
With it, his back straightened
on his full-length matching wooden crutches.
He looked so tall and stately
that my heart almost burst with pride.

Generally, though, he went to work
in his cobbler's shop in town
on a friend's pony and cart,
the left leg of his trousers
neatly tucked around the stump,
emphasizing the loss, but making
its own silent statement about
the indomitable spirit that swung it.

He labored each day in Tralee Market
unselfconscious of the irony
that he was repairing shoes
for the population of the town he loved.
His center was so secure
that he could take the raw leather,
hone it into shape with a sharp knife,
tap-tap-tap it with his hammer
until it was strong and supple;

then, with curled cord, waxed for strength,
he'd sew the moistened strengthened sole
with his awl over the iron last.

It was in that same corner shop
when I was seven
that he sat me on his good knee and,
with wise deliberation,
gave me a puff of his aromatic tobacco pipe.
Much to my mother's outrage
this turned my color green
and made me as sick as any parrot
that ever felt unwell;
but happily it also put me off smoking
for the rest of my life.

His nimble fingers on the button melodeon
also gave me an abiding love of music.
But his real legacy to me was love, not health.
I played hopscotch on the pavement
for hours when he died,
vainly trying to dull the pain of the loss,
hoping to find him again when I landed
on the final square.

I still remember that gentle man
who with his wooden leg stood so tall
that his shadow had the power to protect us all.
I was only ten when he died,
but I still miss my dad.

Reframe the Problem

How can you see a situation differently
so that it becomes a learning
experience rather than
an exercise in blame or guilt?
—Joan Borysenko

When I visit art galleries, I often wonder why the artists or curators chose a particular frame in which to display the painting, and why they chose that particular size and shape rather than another. I once was fortunate enough to ask a painter why she chose to exhibit her portrait of a captain of industry in a square frame. "Because that's his frame of reference, and that's how I see him too—square, solid, and locked into a system."

Solve This Problem

An Arabian chief left his seventeen camels to his three sons. The eldest was to get half, the middle son a third, and the youngest one-ninth. Try as they might they were unable to divide the camels. Finally they went to one of the village elders and asked him for help. He thought for a moment, and then came up with an imaginative solution. When the three sons had finished dividing their camels they thanked the elder and went on their way, happy.

How did the village elder solve the problem? Take some time to figure it out before you read further.

It's very easy to become so immersed in a situation that we become totally blind to the many possibilities for a solution which are always at our disposal. We see only one option and, when that doesn't work out, we consider it a failure and retreat.

But failure is only another name for a "learning experience." When Edison was asked about the number of times he had tried and failed to achieve results, he replied: "Results! Why man, I have gotten a lot of results. I know several thousand things that don't work." After all, as he put it himself, "genius is one per cent inspiration and ninety-nine per cent perspiration."

Reframing a situation is simply looking at it from a different angle, from a new perspective, with a fresh pair of eyes, through green—rather than rose—tinted glasses.

It's been my experience that the answer is always in the original problem. In the work I've been doing over the years with people who come to discuss their life-issues, I've found they benefit enormously from being told: "If you want to know the end, look at the beginning."

What About the Camels?

What's all this got to do with the seventeen camels? Quite a lot. The problem begins with the number of camels. You can't halve an odd number of camels. The village elder knew that, so he reframed the problem. He asked his wife to bring round one of his own camels. When she had done so, he said: "I'm going to give you the gift of a camel. It's yours to keep. The only thing I ask is that, when you've divided up the camels according to your father's wishes, you'd let me have whatever remains." This they agreed to do.

The three sons divided the eighteen camels according to their father's wishes. The eldest, being entitled to half, got nine. The middle son, who was bequeathed one-third, got six. And the youngest, whose inheritance was one-ninth, got two. Now nine, plus six, plus two equals seventeen—precisely the number of camels they were given in the first place! When they had finished laughing at how simple it all was, they returned the extra camel to the village elder and gratefully went back home.

A New Perspective

The secret to reframing is widening our perspective. It means becoming aware that our original frame of reference is too limiting. Sometimes we have to change our standard mind-set and most cherished opinions.

Serious illness necessarily brings with it a whole new frame of reference. If that frame locks us into a pattern of feeling helpless, victimized, and unable to cope, we're going to remain trapped in self-pity until we wake up to the fact that we have to reframe the situation. If the frame locks us into a pattern of welcoming the secondary gains we get from being ill—the sympathy, the attentiveness, and the tender loving care of family and friends—we are effectively going to remain ensnared in a web of unhelpful kindness. This will continue until we're prepared to widen our horizons and begin to take charge of our lives.

A small but useful example of how to reframe involves the use of the Hickman pump. When patients are given chemotherapy at a slow infusion rate via the Hickman line, they have to eat, sleep, go to the toilet, and shower with the pump attached to their body. How do you get a shower in those circumstances? The way I reframed the problem was to get a couple of plastic hooks and superglue them to the shower tiles behind the jet. Now I simply place the pump into a plastic bag and hang it on the hook. There's enough line available to be able to shower front and back with relative ease.

Not An Excuse For Remaining Stuck

Jack was a cantankerous and very uncooperative patient. He also had a wicked sense of humor. One morning the nurse came in and placed a little bottle on top of the trolley at the end of his bed.

"I want you to pass a urine sample into that in your own good time. I'll come back for it later."

"What," exclaimed Jack. "You mean from here?"

Reframing a problem is meant to move us forward to a solution, not become an excuse for doing nothing or keep us firmly rooted in our comfortably familiar groove.

17   Eat Sensibly

*When the body's intelligence is
fully working, then your taste buds
are an excellent guide to
what you should be eating.*
—*Dr. Deepak Chopra*

There are countless books on the market promoting one fad diet after another. The fact is that in the majority of cases these do more harm than good. The whole business of nutrition is really quite simple: all it requires is that you eat healthily and with conscious enjoyment, so that you give yourself enough energy to get through the day. A sensible diet to lose weight means consuming fewer calories than you burn off in a day.

There's still no clear agreement among the scientific and medical communities regarding the link between cancer and what we eat. The latest research indicates that weight gain in later life is a definite risk factor for some cancers. However, from the studies available at present we can indicate some helpful guidelines which are both preventative and restorative.

Many cancer patients undergoing treatment find they are nauseated and do not have much of an appetite for food. However, the nausea can be eased with medication, and a qualified dietician will advise on the best way of regaining lost weight, or of keeping one's weight within limits.

When I first went on steroids all my nausea ceased. I didn't even have to take the anti-nausea pills generally prescribed. However, my eyes were bigger than my tummy. Whenever I looked at the hospital menu, I couldn't resist asking for large portions. I quickly put back on all the weight I'd lost, and even added some more. But I've since learned that more modest meals are better and easier to digest.

Ten Helpful Tips

Here are a few tips which might come in useful. Unless your doctor or dietician has given you a special dietary regime to follow, these guidelines represent the approach of many experts in the field.

1. Don't overeat—take enough to satisfy your hunger but not to the point of bloated fullness. Stop eating when you feel comfortably full. Smaller meals help reduce nausea. Eat when you're hungry. If you have an upset stomach, wait until you're feeling better. Eat your main meal at lunch, not in the evening.

2. Be mindful of every mouthful. Don't eat too quickly, but chew your food well and enjoy the experience. Savor your food, not swallow it. Never eat indiscriminately or on the run. Saying a grace before meals, pausing in thanksgiving for the food, is a good way of slowing yourself down. Don't forget it takes twenty minutes for your stomach to inform your brain that you've had enough.

3. Maintain a high-fiber diet, including whole-grain cereals and plenty of fresh fruit and vegetables, especially those high in the antioxidant vitamins A, C, and E (e.g. cabbage, brussels sprouts, broccoli, cauliflower, and carrots).

4. Lower your fat intake to 30% of your daily calorie needs by cutting down on cheese, eggs, butter, pastries, processed foods, and fatty meats (bacon, sausages, and the like). Give preference to fish and poultry rather than red meat.

5. *Lower your sugar intake.* Sugar actually increases the appetite and leads to overeating.

6. *Avoid alcohol* as much as possible.

7. *Lower your caffeine intake* by not drinking too much coffee, tea , or colas.

8. *Take food that is fresh* and that is cooked for your meal. Avoid reheated leftovers and "junk" food.

9. *Drink about eight glasses of pure water every day.*

10. *Variety is the spice of life.* Eat a well-balanced variety of foods rather than sticking with those few you have been conditioned to since childhood.

18   Cherish Your Friends

*A friend is someone who
knows the song in your heart
and can sing it back to you when
you've forgotten how it goes.*
—Anonymous

When I was growing up in Kerry, in the southwest of Ireland, we used the Irish language, Gaelic, much more frequently than people do now.

When I was thinking about the nature of friendship, an old Gaelic proverb floated back into my consciousness: *Ar scáth a chéile is eadh mhairidh na daoine.* Literally, it means "It's in the shadow of each other that the people live." In other words, we shelter in each other's shadows, we are protected by their presence. And in the barren, windswept landscape of places like the Dingle Peninsula, this took on an added significance.

Friends are essential in all our lives, whether we're healthy or not. There is a barrenness in a life without them. When we don't have friends, there's no one we can absolutely rely on to hold us safe, to sustain us, to provide an umbrella against life's downpours. Effectively we're on our own.

At times of serious illness good friends are vital. They comfort and console us. They're there for us, ready to help in whatever way they can. They may carry around their own emotional and spiritual baggage, but generally they avoid projecting it onto us. Their voice on the phone, their footstep on the stairs, their laughter in conversation, all reverberate within our hearts and play a melody that reminds us that relationships are what life and love are about.

I still remember, after I was told I had cancer, the pain I felt when two close friends of mine didn't visit me in the hospital or even pick up the phone to talk with me for over a month.

It took quite a while for me to realize why. It was not because they didn't value our friendship; it was because they valued it too much.

The fact is that we live in an age when everybody wants to be able to fix things—whether it be a burst pipe or a broken heart. When we can't do so we feel somehow inadequate and, consequently, frustrated.

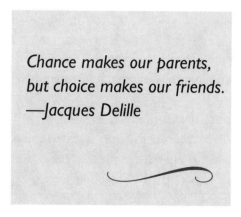

Chance makes our parents, but choice makes our friends.
—Jacques Delille

When my friends were faced with the reality that I had advanced cancer, they knew there was absolutely nothing they could do to fix it. The frustration of having to endure being so ineffective in a time of need, and their determination not to be seen simply mouthing pious nostrums and platitudes, prevented them from coming to the hospital or picking up the phone.

But, it's not what friends *do* for us that matters. It's who they are. It's their shadow, their protective presence that we need. Without saying a word, the mere fact that they care enough to show up speaks volumes. Presents are good, but presence is better.

When we're ill we need to cherish our friends and be understanding of the dilemma in which they sometimes find themselves. We can gently encourage them to come and see us when we feel up to having visitors. It's worth remembering that, much of the time, all friendship requires is that we turn up and gift each other with the protection of our shadow.

19   Maintain Your Sense of Humor

*A cheerful heart is first-rate
medicine; but an unhappy spirit
dries up the bones.*
—*Proverbs 17:22*

There's no situation so desperate that you can't wring humor out
of it. Many people with cancer or another serious illness are noto-
rious for their dark humor. They are somehow able to enjoy a
joke, no matter how close it is to the bone.

*O'Reilly, a poor farmer, dies. His wife, a practical woman, is very upset
and decides to take out an advertisement in the local paper.*

*"I've an advertisement here, with just two words in it—O'Reilly
dead. How much will it cost?"*

"That'll be twenty pounds, Madam."

*"Twenty pounds for just two words! That's ten pounds a word. It's
daylight robbery!"*

*"Well, Madam, our regular advertisements give you five words for
twenty dollars."*

*The farmer's wife thinks about it and finally agrees. The following
day the advertisement duly appears for all to see: "O'Reilly dead. Toyota
for sale."*

Laughter is the Best Medicine
One day, when I was in the middle of writing this book, everything
that could go wrong did go wrong. I started work at 6 a.m. but it
was like pulling teeth to get the words out. Then my computer

71

crashed and I just couldn't find the back-up disk I was looking for. Unexpected visitors called and had to be paid attention to. My energy levels plummeted. I developed a migraine headache and had to go to bed for several hours to relieve it. Definitely a down day! All things considered, what I needed was a good laugh.

That evening I switched on the TV and watched a tribute to the incomparable British comedian, Ken Dodd. He's probably the last of the truly great stand-up comedians who cut their teeth in variety. His humor is anarchically physical, and his obvious enjoyment at being able to make others laugh is infectious. I just sat there and held my "steroid tummy" to ease the pain of the laughter. The relief was incredible. It was like getting a new set of shock-absorbers—it smoothed out the bumps. With his silly antics and machine-gun delivery of original and well-worn jokes and gags, Ken cheered me up. That night I slept like a baby. Without doubt, Shakespeare was right. Sleep knits up "the raveled sleeve of care." But humor is a pullover that warms your heart and keeps you from falling apart.

A sense of humor is a powerful resource when we have to face some of life's greatest difficulties. It gives us a sense of perspective that enables us to gain some emotional distance from our problems and so be in a better position to cope with them.

We need a sense of humor for our physical, emotional, mental, and spiritual health. It's medicine for the soul, a splint to heal our broken places, an injection of life into a tired and weary body. It perks us up when we're physically down and nourishes us when we're emotionally starving. It's a reservoir we can draw sustenance from in times of trouble and distress.

Physically, laughter makes our heart beat faster, increases oxygen in the blood, and has aerobic benefits by shaking our frame and exercising our muscles. When we laugh at our foibles and see the absurdity of our taking things too seriously, we difuse our pain and ease our embarrassment.

Believe it or not, in the stress management field an increasing number of consultants are now teaching executives how to laugh! They're shown how to put a smile on their face and let out a big guffaw or a loud "ha-ha-ha" from their belly.

Naturally, it's a forced reaction at first, and can even be hard work for those who are so poker-faced that they never even break out into a smile, let alone a rib-tickling bout of uncontrollable laughter. But it works. It seems to give people the kick-start they need to appreciate the truth that "we don't laugh because we're happy; we're happy because we laugh."

At an even deeper level, our ability to laugh at ourselves, no matter how dreadful our situation, is ultimately a sign that our spirit transcends the here and now, that this life is not all there is, and that our God will look after us, no matter what may befall us. As Julian of Norwich put it so beautifully: "All shall be well, and all shall be well, and all manner of things shall be well."

There is a good deal of evidence now to suggest that people who can laugh in the face of adversity stand a better chance of recovery than those who cannot. A sense of humor jolts us out of our habitual

> *A smile is a curve that can set things straight.*
> —Anonymous

mind-set and opens up new perspectives. The human spirit cannot be imprisoned in the present or incarcerated in the past. Essentially, it is unrestricted and destined for immortality. In reality, humor is one of the powerful signs or "rumors" of the existence of God.

Hair Loss

A cancer patient on chemo goes into the barber's shop. He's completely bald, except for three hairs on the top of his head.

"A wash, shampoo, and blow-dry, please."

The barber sits him down at the sink and runs the water over the three hairs. But when he's putting on the shampoo, one of the hairs comes away.

"I'm terribly sorry, sir, but I've bad news for you. I'm afraid one of your hairs has fallen out."

"Ah, don't worry about that," says the customer. "When you're finished, just part the other two in the middle."

So the barber continues with the job, but, just as he's using the dryer, a second hair falls out.

"I'm dreadfully sorry, sir, but I'm afraid I've more bad news for you. Another hair has just fallen out."

"Don't worry," says the customer. "When you've finished with the blow-dryer, just leave it tossed!"

A Sick Husband

A woman took her husband to the doctor and asked him to give him a thorough examination. The doctor did so and then took the woman aside to have a quick word with her.

"I don't like the look of him," he said, mournfully.

"Neither do I," said the woman, "but he's very good to the kids!"

A Problem Child

A woman stormed into the doctor's office, dragging her young son by the scruff of the neck.

"I just want to ask you one question, doctor," she said. "Can a boy of ten take out his own appendix?"

"Definitely not, madam," said the doctor.

So the woman gave her son a clip on the ear. "Did you hear that, Jimmy? Now, put it back at once!"

A Couple of Weeks to Live

Maguire was given just two weeks to live, so he told the doctor he'd take one week in January and the other one in July.

20 Listen to Music

*Alas for those who never sing, but
die with all their music in them.*
—Oliver Wendell Holmes

One of the most significant pieces of music in my life has been Pachelbel's *Canon in D.* Every time I listen to it, it moves me. It slows me down, grounds me, and calms my spirit. It touches a chord deep within me that opens my heart to beauty and wonder and compassion.

Music therapy is now a recognized form of healing. Many surgeons regularly ask their patients what music they'd like to hear in the operating room. They know it helps them calm their fears and that it brings an element of the familiar into an otherwise stressful situation.

Music lowers our tension, increases our relaxation response, and gives us a sense of well-being. It does this by engaging the creative right side of our brain. We all differ in the type of music we like. It doesn't matter whether we prefer classical or pop. Sometimes we'll be ready for Bach and at other times the Beatles. Indeed, many people today are rediscovering the power of the ancient rhythms and cadences of plainchant to transform their mood and gently ease their pain.

A good tip if you're a patient is to bring your own personal stereo, headphones, and favorite music into the hospital with you. Listening to soothing music for ten to fifteen minutes can help relax you thoroughly. Through it, you will find a peaceful, contented, and tranquil space to be in. In fact, music is good medicine, because it helps people heal.

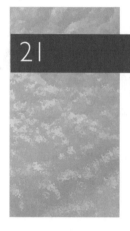

21   Take Regular Exercise

Whenever the urge
to exercise comes over me,
I lie down and wait for it to pass.
—W.C. Fields

It may seem strange to suggest that people with a serious illness should try to keep fit. But it's vital nonetheless. The fitter we are, the more likely we are to improve our chances for getting better quicker.

When their health is reasonably good, many people think exercise is simply a waste of time. As Henry Ford put it: "Exercise is bunk. If you are healthy you don't need it; if you are sick you shouldn't take it!"

But this is a very short-sighted attitude. Exercise brings with it many benefits, not least the fact that it's a way of socializing, of relaxing, and of enjoying the moment. Indeed, in the long term, a lack of proper exercise will inevitably deplete our energy levels and lower our general well-being.

It has now been well documented that exercise strengthens our immune system, increases our cardiovascular efficiency, helps prevent coronary heart disease, aids in reducing high blood pressure, lessens our chances of developing sedentary diseases, burns off calories, aids our concentration, improves our mood, boosts our self-confidence, helps us relax, improves our digestion, keeps our joints supple, gives us improved muscle tone, and even improves our sex lives!

It also increases our stamina, and this can be a tremendous help in coping more effectively with the demands which any serious illness makes on our body.

With all these benefits, is it any wonder that it's recommended for our general health and well-being?

Suitable Forms of Exercise

It's important, however, for those of us who are ill not to get involved in the more competitive forms of exercise. That only serves to raise our tension levels and is simply counterproductive, especially if at the end of it we're tense, upset, or distressed.

The best forms of activity for those who are ill, but are still capable of exercising, are: brisk walking, swimming, tennis, and dancing. It's always a wise move to consult your doctor before undertaking some unaccustomed exercise. Certainly you should do so before you consider jogging or other more strenuous workout sessions.

It's worth noting that even short periods of regular exercise help improve the functions of heart, muscles, and circulation. Even fifteen minutes five times a week will prove to be beneficial. This can eventually build up into a half-hour session. The important thing is to incorporate it into our daily routine so that it becomes a lifestyle choice.

Motivation can be a powerful incentive here. Dog owners, for example, often force themselves to take regular exercise whether they like it or not. They might not be willing to do it for themselves, but they'll do it for their pet!

> *I like long walks, especially when they are taken by people who annoy me.*
> —Fred Allen

Exercise, though, should be an enjoyable experience, not a burdensome chore. That's why it's sensible to choose a form of exercise that makes us feel good and that we enjoy. This will also ensure that we'll continue with it, no matter what the other demands on our time might be.

*If imagination can enhance healing
during times of crisis, it can be just
as effective in health maintenance
and prevention of illness.*
—*Bruce G. Epperly*

One morning, in order to get an early start on this section of the book, I got up at 5 a.m. and went downstairs to get myself something to eat. I opened the refrigerator and found a large lemon on the shelf. Normally I take some grapefruit if I want to stimulate my tastebuds, but this particular morning I wanted to really wake myself up. So I cut the chilled lemon in two and squeezed the ice-cold bitter juice into my mouth, letting it swish around before swallowing it. Then I took the other half and began to squeeze that...

Just stop for a moment. As you've been reading, something has been happening to your body. Usually when I tell this story at workshops, most of the participants find that they've been producing an increasing amount of saliva in their mouths. The mere thought of a cold, juicy lemon at five in the morning is enough to produce the saliva, automatically. Naturally, the story about the lemon is just an invention. I never squeezed a bitter lemon that early in the morning, but it does help illustrate the power the mind has over the body.

Mind/Body Link
Our minds are incredibly creative and resourceful. We can create vivid pictures of absent objects and respond to them as if they were really present. If we imaginatively light a log fire, we can

soon imagine that we begin to smell the smoke. If we imagine we are lying on a beach with the sunlight warming our body, we can even begin to feel the sand under us and find that our body actually warms up.

The fact is that we respond physically and psychologically to the images we create or keep in our mind. This is why we talk about the power of mind over matter. The so-called "placebo" effect is a well-known example. The link between the mind and body is also the reason why visual imagery is now seen as such a powerful tool for healing people.

The good news is that we can use this image-making ability of ours to help manage our moods, redirect our thoughts, relax our muscles, ease our pain, and refresh our spirits.

This powerful tool has been known for thousands of years. It's probably why Hippocrates, the Greek physician who lived five centuries before Christ, said that he would much prefer to know the kind of person who had a disease rather than know what disease the person had.

One of the world's leading experts on the subject, Dr. Carl Simonton, reports that patients using imagery have experienced fewer side-effects and recovered more quickly than those who have not. He has even suggested that, if we're unable to do physical exercise, we should at least imagine ourselves doing it, and that this will give us at least some of the benefits associated with the real thing.

Today the practice of visualization is at the center of many cancer recovery programs throughout the world. On the following pages I've outlined a sample visualization script that you might find useful in your own recovery and healing, or as a help to someone you know.

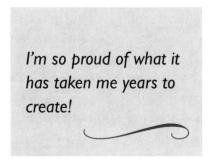

I'm so proud of what it has taken me years to create!

23 Healing Light Visualization

A person's mind stretched to a new idea never goes back to its original dimensions.

The following script is a "Healing Light" visualization specially devised for patients with cancer. It can easily be adapted to any other illness, with equally positive effects.

You can always buy a tape with this material ready to play. But if you prefer, you could speak the words of the conversation into a tape recorder yourself. When you're thoroughly relaxed you could then just switch on the tape and listen to it, following the sequence in your imagination, making the words and images as graphic and real as you possibly can. Each time you do this exercise it becomes more powerful.

To begin this visualization, choose a warm quiet place where you will be undisturbed for about twenty minutes. Close your eyes and let your breathing become rhythmic and deep. Let go of all tension in your body and be aware of how relaxed and calm you're becoming. Count down from ten to one slowly and, as you count, allow yourself to go deeper and deeper into relaxation.

When you're feeling comfortably relaxed, decide to go in your mind to a favorite spot, some place where you can totally relax and be at peace. It might be lying on a beach, or in a meadow, or in a comfortable hotel bed. What matters is that you're there and are completely at rest.

Now, imagine your spirit leaving your body and looking down from the heavens at yourself, lying there, completely relaxed. There is behind your spirit a wonderfully clear white light. It is your helper. Look at yourself lying there, comfortably relaxed. Then, instantly, let your spirit and the white light behind it go straight down and into your body, locating itself in whatever place your cancer happens to be. The light illuminates the area, and you can clearly see the tumor and the lesions and whatever cancerous growth is present. At this point you can speak to your cancer cells as follows:

I want to thank you for the good you have done for me by multiplying so rapidly.

You have given me a real wake-up call. You have reminded me of my mortality. You have made me face up to the reality of death.

You have focused my body, mind, and spirit into getting my priorities straight, clarifying my goals, practicing my beliefs, adhering to my values, and taking my spirituality seriously.

You have challenged me to face up to my responsibilities, acknowledge my interdependence, listen to my body, access my coping skills, widen my horizons, and remain ever open to the wisdom of the infinite mystery that is God's love for me.

I want to thank you for all of this, because, without your activity, I'd probably still be stuck in the same rigid patterns I've developed over the years to protect my fragile ego.

But I now have to tell you that you are actually endangering the very body that has given you life and sustenance. You are putting at risk the host that has supplied the materials for your energy needs. So, your uncontrolled expansion has to stop. You must cease to multiply. This is for the greater good of the whole organism.

To help you do this in a completely painless and effective manner, I'm sending the white light and energy of God into every area of my body where any cancer cells are active. As soon as the light touches these cells, they will immediately stop all activity and will simply melt into the light. This will mean they will have been absorbed into God's infinite energy and will then be able to expand as much as they desire in God, but not in my body.

My body will then be able to heal quickly and be free of its cancer. Every organ will be healed and every lesion and tumor disappear, never to return. I can then get on with my life, having learned the valuable lessons that you have taught me. I can then become a more caring and spiritually aware person as a result of this whole experience.

As the white light of God's energy bathes you in its warmth, you will feel no pain or discomfort as you shrink and grow smaller, until you're eventually incorporated completely into the light.

As you leave, I want to thank you once more. One day, when I've lived my life to the full, we shall meet again and share the light of God's love together. But for now, I wish you goodbye.

When you've finished this conversation, allow some time for the light to bathe the cancer cells. See them shrinking before you and eventually disappearing altogether. When you're ready, you can count up from one to ten, continuing to remain relaxed. However, at the count of ten you will open your eyes and be wide awake and thoroughly refreshed. Just wriggle your fingers and toes, and if you've been lying down, take all the time you need to get up gently.

> *In the midst of winter I discovered within me an invincible summer.*
> *—Albert Camus*

Learn to Say "No"

Tell him to live by yes and no—
yes to everything good,
no to everything bad.
—William James

It has been said that you can divide people into three types: those who can count, and those who can't. (If you didn't get it, I'm not going to explain it!)

I prefer to talk about dividing people into two types: those who automatically say "Yes" when you ask them to do something, and those who automatically say "No."

Life on Automatic Pilot

The problem is that both types are living life on automatic pilot. The reaction they reach for is outside their conscious control. It's as if it were "hard-wired" into their neurological pathways.

Most of us were brought up to believe that the three-letter word "Yes" was somehow better and more virtuous than the two-letter word "No." "Yes" was seen to be something positive, "No" was negative. In reality, of course, the distinction is far more subtle than that. "No" can be an appropriate and positive response at times, while "Yes" can be a cop-out, capitulation, or fearful response to an unjustified demand.

Saying "Yes" compulsively—not wanting to offend or wanting to be seen as a helper or rescuer—is just as bad as saying "No" compulsively. Our responses are only meaningful if we are free to choose.

The sign of a mature personality is the inner freedom to be able to say "Yes" or "No" as appropriate in the circumstances. Our "Yes" has no real value if we are not free at the same time to say "No."

What has all this to do with being seriously ill? A lot, in fact. When people are ill there are enough pressures on them without having to take on the burden of added responsibilities. Family and friends can, without realizing it, put patients in a no-win situation or face them with a moral dilemma they find hard to deal with. It has taken me a long time to learn this and I'm still just finding my way. Let me give you an example.

Some time ago two close friends of mine, Diana and Alan, phoned me from England and asked if they could come over to Dublin to see me during their school's mid-term break. When I inquired about the dates and found they would conflict with the deadline for this book, I surprised both them and myself by issuing an emphatic "No." I knew I had to continue working without interruption if the book were to be published on time. I explained this and we arranged for another, more suitable date.

Afterwards, however, I found myself trying to process the guilt I felt at having to say "No" to two good friends. This, in spite of knowing that my response was actually a positive step towards completing my project.

Visiting Hours

In a hospital situation it's often possible to be inundated with visitors. No matter how happy you are to see them, too many visitors at a time can drain you of energy. Far better for them to space out their visits so that you have someone every evening, rather than a glut of faces on one particular day. This is when the word "No" becomes vitally important. It's a form of self-protection and a positive response to what could otherwise be a stressful situation.

One of the key pieces of advice that therapists and counselors receive during their training is the motto: *when all else fails, protect yourself.* One of the ways of doing this is to have the courage to say "No." It's advice which anybody with a serious illness would do well to adopt.

When we're free to say "Yes" without guilt and "No" without resentment, we're no longer reacting compulsively and we're in a better position to devote what energy we have to our recovery and well-being.

> **I don't know the key
> to success, but the key to failure
> is to try to please everyone.**
> **—Bill Cosby**

25　Keep It Simple

*The person who has a "why" to live
can bear with almost any "how."*
—*Friederich Nietzsche*

Albert Einstein, a sophisticated thinker if ever there was one, once said: "We should keep things as simple as possible—but no simpler!"

This is good advice when dealing with the practical problems that come up for those who have to cope with cancer or another serious illness. In fact, the *KISS* solution is based on it. At stress management workshops I often tell people to kiss their problems away. When they come back for an explanation, all I have to do is spell out the message, *Keep It Simple, Stupid!*

Let's see how it might work in practice.

Doctors/Nurses

Remember your medical team is there to help you. Always treat them with courtesy and try to take into account that there are other patients who also need their attention. A little patience goes a long way. But there's no need to be a mouse either. Tell the doctor clearly what is wrong. Don't minimize your symptoms, but don't exaggerate them either. Be open and up front. This implies not taking unprescribed medication or remedies without clearing this with your doctor first.

Surgery

An operation is always a major event in a person's life. Express how you feel. If you're worried or scared, say so. Fear of the unknown is a real problem, so establish a rapport with your doctor and get the concrete information you need. Consider all the options; there may or may not be an alternative to surgery. Your doctor will be able to advise you on this. Before the operation relax as much as you can.

Pain

It's very much a given that you're going to feel some pain for the first few days after an operation, but if you remember that the pain will lessen before too long and that it can be managed effectively with medication, you will be in a better position to cope.

Chemotherapy/Radiation Therapy

Depending on the nature of your illness, your doctor may prescribe either chemotherapy or radiation therapy or both. It's well to know that others have been through the experience before you and have dealt with it well. Both treatments have potential side-effects but, as we have already noted, we're all different and respond to treatment in different ways. Some people have very little trouble with side-effects, but even if you do, there are counter-remedies for practically everything you are likely to experience. Nausea, for example, can be treated with a variety of different pills, fatigue can be relieved with steroids, and weight loss can be dealt with by the dietician. Any hair loss, which doesn't always happen, is generally temporary, and women, in particular, successfully manage to deal with it by using a wig.

The bottom line is that the benefits of the treatment generally outweigh its unpleasantness, and almost all side-effects are temporary and gradually cease when the treatment is completed.

The angels keep their ancient places
Turn but a stone and start a wing.
'Tis we, 'tis our estrangèd faces
That miss the many-splendored thing!
—Francis Thompson

Most of us are control freaks. We earnestly seek to cover all the bases, spot all the angles, and avoid all the pitfalls.

But the fascinating thing about life is how unruly it is, how unpredictable, how unforeseeable. Just when I think I have my own illness down pat, something totally unexpected happens. Its progression is constantly surprising me. It forces me to acknowledge that I am no longer totally in control, and maybe never was.

I continue to be a participant in my recovery. I continue to take charge of my choices, but essentially I am in other hands—the loving, caring, and tender hands of God, and the experienced, gentle yet strong hands of the nurses, doctors, and consultants who care for me. It has forced me to face up to the truth that God is the one who is ultimately in control. God will take good care of me.

Flexibility and the ability to let go are corollaries of this. They are indicators of our belief in God's loving providence. Strength does not always mean meeting events or problems head-on. Sometimes that smacks more of stubbornness than of street-smarts. Courage frequently involves the decision to cut our losses and live to fight another day. Trees that bend in the wind do not usually break; they flourish when the storm is over.

Unfortunately, flexibility is very difficult for those of us who are over-achievers or continually in control mode. What illness and suffering do is offer us a pathway strewn with unexpected twists and turns, so much so that we cannot presume to know what will happen next. It forces us to put our trust in Someone greater than ourselves. As Isaac Bashevis Singer put it: "Life is God's great novel. Let him write it."

Be Open to the Appearance of the Infinite

Most of us tend to sleepwalk through life. Paul warns us about that: "Now is the time to awake from sleep" (Romans 13:11). Waking up is a sign of maturity, a mark of growth. It is also a proof that we're in touch with what is really real, the depth of things rather than their surface. Essentially, it is the beginning of wisdom.

We are reminded of this in the delightful story of the disciple who went to the Zen master and asked if there was anything he could do which would help him gain enlightenment. The master replied: "Do just as much as you would do to make the sun rise in the morning and set in the evening." But this did not satisfy the disciple. "What's the point, then, of practicing the spiritual exercises you have assigned to me?" The master looked at him with compassion and said gently: "To make sure you are not asleep when the sun begins to rise."

There are "rumors" or traces of God's presence in the most unexpected places, people, and events. God's angels continually guard, guide, and protect us. They remind us we are loved unconditionally and that we are kept ever safe in the palm of God's hand.

Sometimes we turn to God when our foundations are shaking only to find out it is God who is shaking them.
—Anonymous

27   Pray As You Can

If you are too busy to pray,
you are too busy.
—Anonymous

The hospital chaplain was visiting an elderly woman and agreed to pray with her so that she might make a speedy recovery to good health.

"Dear God," he began, "if it is your will to restore Mrs. Doyle to her former health..."

As he was praying he felt a tug on his arm, so he stopped in mid-sentence.

"Excuse me, Father," said the old lady, "but I'd be grateful if you'd call me Lizzie. He won't know me by my married name!"

There's a very wise piece of advice which I've found very helpful in my own life. It comes from Dom Chapman: "Pray as you can," he used to say, "not as you can't."

When we're ill, we're often in no mood for praying. The words just won't come out, the experience we're undergoing is so traumatic that all our energies are devoted to dealing with it. There's nothing left in the tank. Or so we think.

The fact is that we can pray without words. We can make the connection with the divine in an instant and say more with our silence than we ever could with our speech. And that connection will give us energy. Alexis Carrel, the French biologist and Nobel Prize winner, said: "Prayer is a force as real as terrestrial gravity. It

supports us with a flow of sustaining power in our daily lives."
Here are two prayers to help when you're ill.

A Prayer in Times of Trouble

Dear God,
There are times when I feel
so lonely and afraid.
This happens especially
when I'm in pain, or so worried
that I cannot even think straight.

I don't want to die
without ever really having lived.
Help me to cope
in these difficult moments,
and to draw strength from
the support of family and friends.

Grant me some relief right now
from my pain and loneliness
and feelings of vulnerability,
so that they may never cause me
to lose sight of the bigger picture.

Help me today to bear
this heavy burden of illness,
and let my wounds be for me
a path to healing and inner peace.
Above all, help me not to lose hope,
but always to trust
that you love me and care for me,
as do my family and friends.
I make this prayer with all my heart. Amen.

A Cancer Patient's Prayer

Dear God,
I thank you for the gift of life and for my body,
which is so wonderfully made.
Unfortunately, things have somehow
gone wrong and I now have cancer.
Help me to understand that this is no fault
of mine, but one more fact of life to deal with.

Help me to accept my cancer as a wake-up call
to put first things first, to deepen my spirituality,
and to open my heart ever wider to
the wonder of your creation all around me.

I thank you for the comfort and support
of family and friends at this time.
Bless them for the many practical
expressions of love they show me each day.

Help me to ask for what I need and
to be grateful for what is given.
I ask you especially to guide and protect
all the doctors, nurses, and care staff
who look after me.

If it be in my best spiritual interests
I pray that I may be completely cured.
But, most of all, I ask for the gift
of inner healing and peace of mind.
This is my heartfelt prayer today. Amen.

I'm a sucker for love.
I could be bribed by a sardine.
—St. Teresa of Avila

When we're ill we need to be very good to ourselves. In particular we're challenged to love ourselves. Love is the most powerful force in the universe. If anything can help us heal, love will. Not only that, but we'll never be able to express our love for others if we do not first love ourselves. Here are a few practical, down-to earth ways in which we can be good to ourselves.

Plan Occasional Breaks
It's always good to have something to look forward to, especially when you're on long-term treatment. It helps to keep you going when the going gets tough.

Every few months I now schedule something special. Six months into my chemotherapy I told the oncologist I'd always wanted to see the Giant's Causeway in Northern Ireland before I died and that I was in fact going the following month, no matter what happened. He was pleased I was so positive, so off I went with a close friend of mine, traveled along the stunningly beautiful Antrim coastline, stayed locally, and enjoyed one of the wonders of the world formed some fifty million years ago.

Accept the Gifts that Come Your Way
One of the secrets of living in the moment is the ability to be

open to the unexpected. When I went to the Giant's Causeway I thought *that* was going to be the highlight of my visit to Northern Ireland. But it turned out that a visit to Bushmills Distillery, the oldest licensed distillery in the world, was much more fun. When we'd been shown how the whiskey was made, we were all shepherded into the bar. The guide called for four volunteers and I immediately put up my hand and was chosen. She asked us to sit at a specially prepared table, with ten tumblers of whiskey in front of us. Six were blended, and four were single malt. This was a tasting session and we were expected to sip each one and say which of the blended whiskeys we preferred and which of the malt.

Of course, I wasn't born yesterday. Neither were the three other volunteers. We all picked Irish whiskeys (as opposed to Scotch and American) and the guide was suitably impressed. She congratulated us and left us for a few minutes. When she returned, she presented us with special certificates inscribed with our names. So, you're now reading material written by a certified Irish whiskey drinker!

But the fun part is that, although I rarely drink more than a half dozen times in the year, like the other volunteers I then proceeded to polish off all ten sample glasses, grab hold of my friend, and float out of the distillery with a smile on my face that would have cheered even a pessimist's heart.

Give Yourself a Treat

Depending on how you're feeling and how mobile you are, this could range all the way from a week's holiday abroad to a candlelit dinner for two in a good restaurant. The point is that you're taking practical steps to pamper and be good to yourself, and this will inevitably make you feel good, lighten your spirits, and assist your body to recover its lost energy.

Welcome the Healing Touch

As any child will tell you when a mother cradles her in her arms, there is comfort and support and healing in good human touch. Handshakes, hugs, kisses, and caresses are all conveyors of affection and love.

When we're ill we need the assurance and consolation of close human contact. A healthy person needs at least one good hug a day. Someone who is ill needs two. And those of us with cancer or another serious illness need at least three!

I was very fortunate during my initial long stay in the hospital to see the power of touch in action. Ken, who was in the bed opposite me, was doing very poorly. He was the most distressed person in the ward and we all ached for him. His wife, Cecilia, used to come in twice a day and sit with him for hours. Sometimes she would read to him, sometimes when he'd drifted off she would doze or pray or read to herself. But always she was there.

One day I happened to be looking at them when Ken was having great difficulty breathing. What happened next took only a couple of moments, but for me time stood still. I saw his hand rise just a little, anchored by his elbow. Immediately, and with great tenderness, Cecilia placed her right hand under his and her left on top of it to tell him she was there. This loving gesture was so comforting that, imperceptibly, the hands dropped back on to the bed and Ken once more drifted into a comfortable sleep. I thought my heart would break at the tenderness of this visible sign of love, this rumor of angels, this gift of making the invisible visible. The infinite was in our midst in that sacred moment. It has stayed with me ever since and been a source of strength and comfort when things have been going badly.

Cultivate a Flower

Men's wards and women's rooms in the hospital are very different. Usually in women's rooms you find vases of flowers and displays of cards, and there's generally more a feeling of home about the place. Men's rooms, by contrast, tend to be bare and a bit spartan. The gentle touch is often missing.

One morning I woke up with an overpowering desire to keep something alive in the ward while I was there. I wheeled my chemo trolley out and found an abandoned carnation. Its stem was broken and it had been left for dead. I retrieved it, cut the stem with a scissors and put it into a small vase of water. For the rest of my stay I continued to care for it.

Since that day I've always had a flower in my room. I water it every day and it reminds me that, in order to flourish, I need to nourish myself too. This reminder is a necessary part of my recovery, and I'm grateful for the opportunity to look after my flower.

Make an Album or Scrapbook
Memories help keep the heart alive. Looking through a photo album of the places you've been or the enjoyment you've had with family and friends, brings a warm glow to the spirit. Enjoy the experience and keep adding to the memories.

> *One who wants a rose must respect the thorn.*
> —*Persian Proverb*

Howard and Mollie are close friends of mine. While I was in the hospital I got a marvelous poster of their grandchildren from them. They'd printed it from the family computer, colored it, and sent it off to me. It was about three feet long, but when I saw it, and the message: "Get Well Soon," I knew I had to find a place for it. I went along to the nurses' station, got some adhesive and stuck it on the wall over my bed. Then I got all my cards and put them up around it. The others thought I'd gone mad. But, guess what? Nobody who visited our ward passed by without joyfully commenting on the poster and reiterating its sentiments. I can't tell you how good it made me feel.

Count Your Blessings

There's always something to be thankful for in life. It's amazing how many things we can find to be grateful for when we try. When I was first diagnosed with cancer, I started a gratitude diary. I called it "My Thank You, God, Diary." I bought a half dozen small notebooks with yellow covers. Every evening I write down briefly, in two or three lines, five things I've found that I'm grateful for that day. Not only does this keep my daily focus positive and make me feel good, but I now have trouble choosing which five items to include. There are always many more which I have to leave out!

Spend Some Time in Meditation

We've already spoken about prayer and spirituality and about the technique of visualization. Meditation can be either secular or religious. It can help calm our "monkey mind" which is distracted and all over the place. But it can also draw us into our center, where we can connect with our real selves and with the divinity present within us. This can be a transforming experience and lead to deep inner peace.

Let Your Inner Child Out

Many of us are too uptight for our own good. We need to lighten up and let go; to let God be God and trust that all shall be well.

When I was first put on steroids and took a break in London with some friends, I acted like a ten-year-old as I dragged them around the shops, enjoying every minute of my new-found energy. I took them to Hamleys in Regent Street—five floors of toys, games, magic, and wonder. I reveled in the joy of it, bought some funny hats and some magic tricks, and generally had a whale of a time. I can still access the memory of that visit and it cheers me up just to recall it.

There are too many dead people walking around today. Dead emotionally, psychologically, and even spiritually. Many people are dead at forty and are only given a decent burial at eighty. Children know how to live life to the full, how to be in the moment, how to look with the eyes of wonder, and marvel at what is, simply because it is there. That's why it makes sense to let our inner child out.

Talk it Out
A trouble shared is a trouble halved. When we learn to talk about our anger, fear, guilt, depression and even despair, we're no longer completely in their power. It's also important to talk about the things we care about with the people who matter most to us. My first cousin died many years ago of a terminal disease. His wife told me recently that, two years before he died, his voice went and he couldn't speak. Ever since then she's regretted the fact that they were never able to speak about their love for each other. So, be good to yourself and learn to talk it out. This is how we heal.

29 Accept the Reality of Death

*Even though I move
through a dark valley, I fear no harm.
For you are beside me with your rod
and your staff to give me courage.*
—Psalm 23:4

Each one of us has a song to sing. We may not have a note in our head or be able to hold a tune. That does not matter. For the song we have to sing is in our heart, not our mouth. Nobody else on this earth can sing it for us. If we pass through this life without having sung it, the world and everybody in it, including ourselves, will be the poorer for it.

But if we discover the song in our heart and express it to the best of our ability, we will enrich our world and, no matter whether our lives are long or short, our living will not have been in vain. When it is time for us to leave it, the world we lived in will be a better place. Our life's task will have been completed and we will be able to go home to God peacefully and rest in Infinite Love.

Jeanie's Song

Jeanie was one of the most loving people I have ever met. She lived to express her love. I first got to know her when her younger sister Anne married my brother Liam. She radiated warmth, affection, and genuine compassion for people, especially for her extended family and the students she taught.

Some years ago she died. They told me she was close to death, but I was already committed to workshops and couldn't cancel at short notice without seriously disrupting many people's lives. Five days later, on a Sunday, I was free. She was still alive. I made the five-hour journey to get to her bedside and say goodbye. When I got there I was shocked. She was so emaciated and her breathing was difficult. I found it very difficult to see her like that. It was obvious that she was still clinging on to life. I wondered was it for people like me to have an opportunity to say goodbye in person.

Her sister was there and told me one of my nephews had said: "Jeanie was my inspiration." Another nephew of hers had flown in from London to be at her bedside. He had left his classes at the London School of Economics to be there. I noticed he had his hand under the blanket and was gently holding hers. I told him how good he was to come all that way and he looked at me in surprise before saying: "I'd have come from the ends of the earth for Jeanie."

I nearly lost it then. I was so close to breaking down in a flood of self-pitying tears. But the closeness of death has a way of forcing us to face up to a dimension of our lives that we sometimes gloss over. So, as I sat there at her bedside, I meditated on my own death and asked myself some very important questions.

When I come to die, will anybody say of me that I was their inspiration? Will anyone hold my hand under the blanket to remind me of the presence of love? And will anyone say that they'd come from the ends of the earth to be with me at my last moments? At the time I couldn't answer "yes" to any of these. But Jeanie could, because she had sung her love-song. The following day she died, peacefully.

Death is a fact of life which we all have to face up to and accept. We cannot ignore its magnitude. Too many people are so afraid of this reality that they choose to live as if they were never going to die. They prefer to remain on the surface, floating on life's ocean without plumbing its depths. They are content with the distractions of superficial living and so never succeed in finding their own unique voice. Their song is locked deep within, hidden even from themselves.

It's only when we accept the fact of our mortality that we can truly learn to live.

> *I have met death, but now I'm alive;*
> *and I shall live for eternity.*
> *—Revelation 1:18*

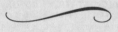

Celebrate Life

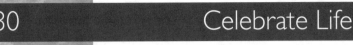

> *There is no cure*
> *for birth and death*
> *save to enjoy the interval.*
> —George Santayana

The best way to prepare for the inevitable reality of death is to celebrate the gift of life.

When we Irish raise our glasses in a toast during a celebration we say *Sláinte,* which literally means "health." There are similar sounding words in other languages, with the same meaning (*Salud* in Spanish; *Salute* in Italian and *Santé* in French). In English we have the rather insipid *Cheers.*

We Irish, of course, are noted for our wakes, where the life of the deceased is toasted in song and story as well as in spirits, especially whiskey, *uisce beatha,* the water of life. But for the best toast of all it's hard to beat the Jews. They really know what life is about and that's why they celebrate it every time they raise a glass and say *l'Chaim,* which literally means "to life."

That's what we should all rejoice in. Not just the life we've had, and not only the life which is to come (even eternal life), but the life we live in the here and now. Our greatest challenge is probably that of saying "Yes" to life, to exult in it and revel in its mystery.

I remember many years ago when the then UN Secretary General, Dag Hammarskjöld, wrote his superb *Markings,* how many people were deeply impressed by his spirituality and his passion for life. In it he wrote movingly about committing him-

103

self wholeheartedly to living, even to the point of being willing to sacrifice himself:

"I don't know Who—or What—put the question. I don't know when it was put. I don't even remember answering. But at some moment I did answer "Yes" to Someone—or Something—and from that hour, I was certain that existence is meaningful and that, therefore, my life in self-surrender had a goal."

Life is dynamic, not static. It's constantly changing, becoming ever new. It abhors stagnation and exults in growth. The sound of the song we sing in our hearts reverberates around the world and influences others for good or ill. When our song is one of love, it energizes us and gives meaning to everything we do.

At the end of his novel *The Bridge of San Luis Rey*, Thornton Wilder tellingly makes this point. He writes: "There is a land of the living and a land of the dead, and the bridge is love, the only survival, the only meaning."

Of course, there's a price to be paid for all this. In life, as in politics, there's no such thing as a free lunch. The price we pay is the selfless leap of faith that Dag Hammarskjöld speaks about, that willingness to walk out into the unknown, trusting in the belief that Love is at its center.

In the Bible, the first words God spoke in the book of Genesis were: "Let there be light." In effect what God was saying was: "Let there be life." And there was life. In the epilogue to the book of Revelation at the end of the Bible, the Spirit says: "Let those who are thirsty come; let all who want the water of life have it as a free gift."

Life is for living, and the only time to live is now. *L'Chaim!*

A Final Story

At the beginning of the book I said that I loved stories. I've tried my best to incorporate many of them in the text to illustrate the points being made. Here's one about St. Francis of Assisi which I like very much and which puts what I've written in context.

Francis and Brother Juniper were out walking one day. They went into the forest and walked for miles until they were very hungry. Eventually Juniper began to get anxious, but Francis reassured him that all would be well.

Just then, they came upon a clearing in the forest, with a small wooden shack at one end. Smoke was coming from the chimney and, as they drew closer, they noticed a large sign outside the shack. It simply said: "Fresh Bread Baked Here Every Day."

Francis looked at Juniper as if to say: "I told you so. The Lord always provides." Then he knocked on the door and it was opened by an old

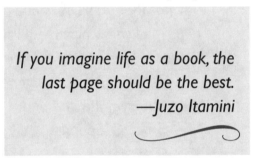

If you imagine life as a book, the last page should be the best.
—Juzo Itamini

woman. She greeted them warmly and asked if she could help.

Francis said: "We'd be very grateful for some of your fresh bread, please."

The woman's face fell, and she looked at the two hungry travellers with sympathy.

"I'm very sorry," she said, "but here we only make the signs!"

That's all this book does too. It gives pointers, tools, techniques and strategies. The rest is up to you. So, this isn't really the end. In reality, like your life, it is only

The Beginning ....

*Physicians are discovering
what their more religious patients
have always known—
that prayer makes a difference
and that difference may be
a matter of life and death.*
—Bruce G. Epperly

Useful Addresses

American Cancer Society National Office
1599 Clifton Road NE
Atlanta, GA 30329
1-800-ACS-2345
www.cancer.org
The Society is a basic resource for information about cancer and its treatment. Printed and audiovisual materials are available to the public, and the toll-free number handles questions and concerns about cancer. Regional, state, and local chapters may provide patient and family education, as well as information, guidance programs, support groups, and practical services.

Cancer Information Service
The National Cancer Institute
Building 3, Room 10A24
9000 Rockville Pike
Bethesda, MD 20892-3100
1-800-4-CANCER
www.cancernet.nci.nih.gov
Cancer Information Service (CIS) serves the entire United States and answers cancer-related questions from the general public, cancer patients and their families, and health professionals. They also offer publications for both patients and health care professionals.

Candlelighters Childhood Cancer Foundation
1312 18th Street NW
Suite 200
Washington, DC 20036
1-800-366-2223
Provides the coordination and educational arm of an international network of self-help groups, along with publications and resources on pediatric cancer.

Make Today Count
101 1/2 S. Union Street
Alexandria, VA 22314
(703) 548-9674
An international organization for persons with cancer or other life-threatening illnesses. Local chapters provide emotional self-help through formal programs, group discussions, newsletters, social activities, workshops and seminars, and educational activities.

National Coalition for Cancer Survivorship
1010 Wayne Avenue Suite 300
Silver Spring, MD 20910
(301) 585-2616
A network of independent organizations and individuals working in the area of cancer support and survivorship, whose primary goal is to generate a nationwide awareness of cancer survivorship.

National Association for Home Care
519 C. Street NE
Washington, DC 20002
(202) 547-7424
Provides information and referral to state associations of licensed home health agencies and a membership directory, along with a pamphlet titled "How to Select a Home Care Agency."

National Hospice Organization
1901 N. Moore Street
Suite 901
Arlington, VA 22209
(703) 243-5900
A Nonprofit organization that provides literature and information about hospice to patients and their families and referrals to local, regional, and national resources.

Select Bibliography

Benson, Herbert. *The Relaxation Response*, Avon, 1975.

_____*Timeless Healing*, Simon & Schuster Ltd., 1996.

Borysenko, Joan. *Minding the Body, Mending the Mind*, Bantam Books, 1988.

Buckman, Dr. Robert. *What You Really Need to Know About Cancer*, Pan Books, 1997.

Cousins, Norman. *Anatomy of an Illness*, W.W. Norton,1979.

Dyer, Wayne W. *You'll See It When You Believe It*, Arrow, 1990.

Epperly, Bruce G. *Spirituality & Health, Health & Spirituality*, Twenty-Third Publications, 1997.

Fitzgerald, Eddie; Bergin, Éilís. *Stress and How to Deal with It*, SDB MEDIA, 1994.

Hanh, Thich N. *Peace is Every Step*, Bantam, 1991.

Kfir, Nira; Slevin, Maurice. *Challenging Cancer: From Chaos to Control*, Tavistock/Routledge, 1991.

LeShan, Lawrence. *How to Meditate*, Bantam, 1974.

Peck, M. Scott. *The Road Less Travelled*, Arrow, 1990.

Pennington, M. Basil. *Centering Prayer: Renewing an Ancient Christian Prayer Form*, Image Books, 1982.

Siegel, Bernie. *Love, Medicine and Miracles*, Arrow, 1989.

_____*Peace, Love and Healing*, Arrow, 1991.

Simonton, O.Carl; Simonton, Stephanie; Creighton, James. *Getting Well Again*, Bantam Books, 1984.

Whitehouse, Michael; Slevin, Maurice. *Cancer: The Facts*, Oxford University Press, 1996.

Weil, Andrew. *Health and Healing:Understanding Conventional and Alternative Medicine*, Houghton Mifflin, 1983.

Of Related Interest...

Wrestling with God and Cancer
A Personal Journey
Beverly Lancour Sinke

The author shares some of her deepest thoughts and feelings, doubts and faith, dark moments and joy-filled ones, as she struggles to understand and live with two harsh realities: the death of her baby and an ongoing battle with cancer. Her honesty and courage, her vulnerability and faith can offer encouragement and hope to those suffering from a serious illness.

ISBN: 0-89622-998-X, 96 pages, $9.95

Cancer and Faith
Reflections on Living with a Terminal Illness
John Carmody

This book contains over forty inspiring and comforting reflections for the terminally ill as they deal with the spiritual and emotional implications of suffering and death. ISBN: 0-89622-594-1, 160 pages, $9.95

The Pummeled Heart
Finding Peace Through Pain
Antoinette Bosco

This touching and amazing story of one woman's struggle to confront many forms of suffering (including a failed marriage, raising and supporting six children alone, and tragic deaths in the family) offers a model of trust and hope in God, and offers encouragement to overcome the difficulties of one's own life.

ISBN: 0-89622-584-4, 140 pages, $7.95

Seeking Inner Peace
The Art of Facing Your Emotions
John Powers

These inspiring reflections help readers to look realistically at their emotions and personality and offers suggestions for achieving balance and peace in one's life.

ISBN: 0-89622-344-2, 112 pages, $8.95

Available at religious bookstores or from:

TWENTY-THIRD PUBLICATIONS
PO BOX 180 • 185 WILLOW STREET (ⓢ) MYSTIC, CT 06355 • 1-800-321-0411
FAX: 1-800-572-0788 BAYARD E-MAIL: ttpubs@aol.com
Call for a free catalog